TO LOVE
AND
TO CHERISH

A continuing relationship with Alzheimer's disease

Katy Samuels

> *If you are continuing
> to travel the road described
> in these pages,
> then I dedicate this book to
> you.*

The front cover picture is of the sycamore tree in the Rectory Garden - taken by Peter. He greatly enjoyed looking at this tree from his Study window.

© Katy Samuels 2015

Introduction

To Love and to Cherish is a natural sequel to my previous book entitled *Order out of Chaos*. In some way I am trying to make sense of this newly created order and to see if it has any impact on my continuing relationship with Alzheimer's disease. I am still left with the slightly ludicrous feeling that everything that has happened is part of the plot of a black comedy. In case you have not read *Order out of Chaos* it may be helpful to present those family members who appear in *To Love and to Cherish*.

The main character is Peter, who has been living with the diagnosis of Alzheimer's disease since the year 2000.

I am Katy and have been married to Peter since 1963. Paul, Rachel and Mark are our three children, born between 1964 and 1969.

Peter and I have six grandchildren, born between 1992 and 2003.

Danny, aged 14, and Alex, 11, are the children of Paul.

Joe, 18, and Amber, 13, are Rachel's children.

Molly, 8, and William, 7, are Mark's children.

The children's ages refer to the year 2010, which is the year of the completion of *To Love and to Cherish*.

Contents **Page**

Chapter One   Some striking contrasts   13

Chapter Two   Questions
                   - but very few answers   35

Chapter Three   Problem solving and thinking
                                              aloud   77

Chapter Four   Testing times   83

Chapter Five   Converting a bed-room
                                 into a bed-sit   89

Chapter Six   Another change of direction   111

Chapter Seven   The unravelling   121

Chapter Eight   Crossroads   125

For Your Own Notes   131

TO LOVE AND TO CHERISH

The Forgotten Body

Unaware of what's before them,
Blind to what's behind,

Stripped of all
emotion,
Lost on the inside.

Missed and mourned for dead,
Though well above their grave.

What is life without a mind?

Just a lost and lonely soul
Wandering high above its body.

The sensitivity and understanding contained in these words, from the mind of Joe, our sixteen year old grandson, may well be what is needed for a relationship with Alzheimer's disease to develop into a continuing relationship. Tangled within the disease and the relationship is the result of the catastrophic loss of the essence of a loved personality. All relationships involve elements of loving and cherishing and the intrusion of Alzheimer's disease in no way reduces the need for those two qualities. But how can such a relationship be sustained? How can the essence of the loved one's personality be preserved when there is the danger, albeit unintentional, of the loved one becoming the subject of care, rather than the unique individual who once enjoyed independence of mind, body and spirit? I am still searching for some sort of answer to this question, but perhaps the words loving and cherishing will provide one or two clues. Perhaps you are involved in a similar search. It may be that you also are struggling to connect a loved one's lost and lonely soul with his or her forgotten body. If you and I are travelling along the same road we may be able to share a few experiences.

As I mentioned in the concluding words of *Order out of Chaos* - which is the book resulting from my two years' work on this whole concept of a relationship with Alzheimer's disease - I have been considering a plan to make some sense of the thoughts and observations contained within the book.

I could repeat many of the points I have already made, but the most significant realisation, from my own point of view, is the pace of the disease. I suspect that an initial response on seeing Peter, after an interval of perhaps a few months, would be that there had been a rather rapid decline in his condition. However, reading through the notes, possibly in batches of three months, might suggest that, rather than the decline being rapid, the decline has followed a systematic and steady path at a relentless but consistent pace. This, in turn, might suggest that the disease has progressed in a calculated and perhaps inevitable manner. Bearing in mind that each individual person will be experiencing symptoms which will be peculiar to that individual, there must still be a general pattern for the progress of the disease. So where does that leave us? Peter is still here but seems unaware of most of the life he is living. From the family's perspective we have realised that accepting what goes on in our house as being entirely normal goes a long way to making what goes on acceptable. Acceptance results in a reduction of frustration and annoyance. Acceptance also helps those charged with his care to continue to love and to cherish that whole person hiding behind the shadow of a forgotten body. The body may have forgotten itself but the carer must take responsibility for remembering all that he was - and so to love and to cherish.

I am considering different ways of continuing the monitoring of Peter's condition and behaviour, and am working on the idea of making a daily comparison - in a very brief way - of the situation on, for example, February 1st 2010, with the situation as recorded on February 1st 2009 and February 1st 2008. This could be recorded on a daily basis which may then give us a clearer idea of what has been going on over the two year period, and may prove to be helpful in understanding the nature of Alzheimer's disease as it is lived in this house.

Chapter One - Some striking contrasts

Monday February 1ˢᵗ 2010

February 2008:
How interesting. I returned from a visit to the hospital and found Peter, at five past three, already dressed and busily engaged in washing up whatever he could find in the kitchen.

On reading this entry for February 2008 I am struck by how much has happened in these last two years. So many skills have been lost.

February 2009:
Peter's reluctance to leave his bed or understand the few simple things required of him - things like sitting up in order to eat his breakfast, or even to swing his legs over the side of the bed in order to sit on the edge of the bed - illustrates situations we are still finding one year later in what we might now call the Project. The Lever Arch File has lost its restraining bar. Readers of the Project will quickly appreciate the significance of this comment.

February 2010:
I changed Peter's pyjama trousers before I went out at eight o'clock this morning. Naturally, he tried to resist with as much vigour as he could muster. Fortunately I mustered a

little more and the operation was successfully carried out. By keeping close to the ground I remained clear of his flapping clenched fists. Needless to say, as soon as the clean trousers were ready to be pulled up over the bottom, the fists ceased flapping and the trousers were hoisted up in a sensible and stylish way. He returned to bed very quickly, leaving me to sort out the morning's agenda. The rest of the day has been quiet and calm, although I think Peter has slept, as opposed to dozed, through a greater part of the day than I would have expected. If Peter can be persuaded to climb upstairs for a bath by half past eleven I shall consider the day to be outstanding, as my great aim in life is to end each day before midnight, instead of in the early hours of the next day. It seems a modest enough ambition! Why should it be beset with difficulties, I wonder??

Tuesday February 2nd 2010

February 2008:
It dawned on me that the presence of another person in the Study with Peter may be a distraction for him. It is possible that he is more able to concentrate on whatever he is doing, or thinking about, when on his own. This would, of course, have been the norm for most of his working life. The Study was his and would generally be occupied by him and him alone. It may not be a brilliant deduction, but is, I am sure, perfectly valid.

February 2009:

I am still looking for signs of new behaviour but, for the time being, the preferred behaviour involves sorting and lining up as much crockery and cutlery as comes Peter's way.

February 2010:

Today's main preoccupation has been with straightening the front door mat and trying to make the bean bags stand to attention. This is a little difficult as it is not in the nature of bean bags to do anything other than flop and respond to the call of gravity.

Wednesday February 3rd 2010

February 2008:

I am very pleased to have been able to turn the clock to February 2008. I can only imagine that my brain must have been in rather better order, as I have recorded some notes which have had a lasting effect on what is happening with Peter and his care, or carer, if there is any difference! I actually wrote that I had been looking at what was happening to Peter as though Peter was the person he used to be. Consequently I had failed to see the more positive sides of life. Peter's grasp on what he had lost had so diminished that the tremendous value of routine, comfort, security in his environment - and the pleasures of a very comfortable bed, together with the ability to sleep for at least eighteen of the twenty-four hours allotted to each day - needed to be placed, most firmly, in the equation. Once that had been established, I was able to see that, in fact, Peter's quality of life was remarkably good and appropriate for the situation in which we all now find ourselves. As you can see, the report for the day was a good one!!

February 2009:
Today's challenges include sorting, folding, reorganising the kitchen and trying to make sense of the presence of four children at the end of the school day. But we have already established a new understanding of our combined mental processes, and can feel certain that Peter is busy doing what his brain is telling him to do. Perhaps my brain will start to tell me what to do - instead of leaving it to my imagination.

February 2010:
I am writing rather earlier than usual today but, so far, the day is progressing very well. Peter has been looking out of the window, but I am not absolutely certain that he is registering the very gentle fall of soft sleet. It falls quite beautifully but is not settling, so perhaps this is a challenge to the mind.

Thursday February 4th 2010

February 2008:
I learnt, through a series of revelations, that it is not necessarily the best idea to try and analyse the meaning of life through the mind gripped by dementia - which is possibly a simple way of recording a chaotic day. *Tempus Fugit* - for which many thanks!!

February 2009:
An excellent day has been recorded. Thank you, Peter.

February 2010:
Peter's day has been excruciatingly quiet and sleepy but, I am thankful to say, he did appear to respond to the sight of Amber's delicious chocolate cookies which she made on coming home from School. Peter may not have been attracted into the kitchen by the wonderful smell of baking, but his eyes did not let him down when he decided to try and organise the chefs out of the kitchen. This must be a very positive sign of good mental health.

Friday February 5th 2010

February 2008:
Extreme restlessness and a marked difficulty in responding to the simplest of gentle requests. At this stage I am beginning to wonder whether or not Peter is more at ease when in a room on his own.

February 2009:
Abandoned buzzing electric razors and taps left discharging expensive metered water have combined to make me reconsider the conservation of the planet's energy - also my own energy. I am going to consider having taps installed which will automatically turn off after a set amount of time.

February 2010:
Peter was wandering round the landing at half past eleven this morning so, in view of my appointment at three o'clock this afternoon, I decided to start the dressing and breakfast process there and then. From then on the day proceeded with incredible ease and simplicity and Peter was not only asleep when I set off for my appointment, but was also asleep, emergency rations uneaten, on my return. The rest of the day was very good. I must mention that, over the last few weeks, Peter has been greatly attracted to the instant coffee jar. Today that attraction proved to be totally irresistible. Peter made himself a drink of coffee. Coffee with two differences. The first one concerns the strength. The dilution was two hundred grammes of coffee to one thirty millilitre - 30ml - measure of warm water. The resulting sticky mass resulted in the second difference. The caffeine-rich liquid was resting in the large coffee jar. It will have to stay in that jar and be measured out by the teaspoon.

Saturday February 6th 2010

February 2008:
This is the first record of not only sorting out the kitchen, but also rearranging furniture, straightening pictures and going on self-conducted tours of the house. Rachel went into hiding in order to complete her work on the laptop. The only obvious difference leading up to Peter's behaviour was the fact that he had not been able to allow himself to go to bed until half past two in the morning and, as a result, would

have been very tired. Does exhaustion lead to over-activity? Not in my case! How about you?

February 2009:
The record claims that there has been a vast transformation in Peter's *modus operandi*. He was very co-operative and appeared to be able to respond to some simple requests. The taps have been changed but the razor continued to buzz after use. Also it has gone on record that Peter was able to use the term, 'Thank you,' appropriately.

February 2010:
Yesterday's early call was not repeated today. Breakfast was not until half past two and the rest of the day has gone on very peacefully. I am presently investigating another communication. For several nights, when sitting in the Study, I have slowly realised that, when Peter fixes me with a puzzled, but still a hard stare, flaps his hands, points to the top of the bookcase facing the window and makes inarticulate sounds, he is actually telling me that he wants his Study to himself. If I leave quietly he settles back in the chair and looks at his chosen reading material - Pevsner's *Cumbria*.

Sunday February 7th 2010

February 2008:
Today has been recorded as a very passive day with Peter not involving himself in very much at all.

February 2009:
When I read last year's contribution it was difficult to believe we were talking about the same person. This year there was no indication of any shred of passivity. But there were many indications of bizarre behaviour which arose, I am sure, from the fact that Peter was quite unable to respond to the signal to get ready for a bath and bed. As a result he spent some long time wandering about, getting colder and colder, because he was only wearing his underclothes. He did not appear to know that he was cold. The day was long and difficult.

February 2010:
This afternoon saw the arrival of the Rapid Response Team - in the form of Rachel and Amber - to assist in a total cleaning programme of the entire house - including washing the paintwork. This is in readiness for a possible curtailing in normal cleaning while my right hand is recovering from Wednesday's carpal tunnel surgery. The team was wonderfully and cheerfully efficient. Peter was very puzzled by the sight of so much industry but managed to escape into the Study for most of the afternoon. Except for the time when the kitchen floor had been washed, of course. I had placed some pieces of newspaper on the floor to enable people to move around in the kitchen. Peter was thrilled because it gave him a wonderful opportunity not only to fold up sheets of paper but also to crawl over the wet floor. He was very pleased. We may not have been pleased but we

were certainly resigned to the inevitability of the situation. So the day has been a good day!!

Monday February 8th 2010

February 2008:
An excellent day.

February 2009:
Although Peter was managing to get out of the bath on his own, and even trying to put on his pyjamas, there was a moment of considerable disorientation which appeared to be because I was in the wrong place at the wrong time. I was still writing in the children's bedroom when he wandered out of the bathroom, and this made it very difficult for him to follow the stages necessary for actually getting into bed. This event would turn out to be another point of reference as far as Peter's care and management is concerned. It is easy to forget how quickly the boat can be rocked!!

February 2010:
A great deal of work has been done in completing the cleaning, washing, cooking, making transport plans for other people and finding substitutes for jobs, but I am still not absolutely certain how I am going to fasten Peter's polished shoes with the fingers of my left hand. Of course it may well be that I return home with more of my right hand exposed than I might have anticipated. But, whatever happens, there is a definite advantage in our particular domestic arrangement - namely the total lack of pressure as

far as time is concerned. I cannot drive for at least seven days so Peter can take as long as it takes to complete any job. He is still efficient with the toothbrush and can manage fairly reasonably with the razor. Food will not be a problem as he is happy to enjoy whatever I place in front of him. Hair washing may have to be rethought, as will separating him from his underpants and trousers. The tie, if it proves to be a challenge, can stay on top of the chest of drawers for a few days. So we shall see if the mental preparation is of any use when the challenge presents itself. The hand operation should be carried out in thirty hours' time - and I can scarcely wait.

Tuesday February 9th 2010

February 2008:
Everything is clear. The record states: Good children and a good Grandad. Which just goes to show . . . something!

February 2009:
Rachel was so eager to report on hearing a few coherent words that she forgot to mention the fact that she had been locked out of the house as a result of Peter having dropped the little catch on the front door. She later advised that I should perhaps take steps to remember to wear a door key round my neck. My retort was to query the nature of the metal used for such an important piece of high fashion. Care would need to be taken to reduce any chance Peter might seize to sabotage the front door.

February 2010:
This time tomorrow the hand will be in good order and all will be well. I can think of little else. Peter has had a good day.

Wednesday February 10th 2010

February 2008:
A very good day is reported.

February 2009:
A year later and Peter is still having a good day.

February 2010:
The carpal tunnel operation was successfully performed this morning. I am hoping for a great improvement as a result of the procedure. It was most interesting to see the whole operation and to be able to listen to the Consultant explain what he was doing. Peter does not appear to have noticed the very large and bulky dressing - which closely resembles a white boxing glove! I am typing with my left hand - and will definitely have to use the spell-checker to highlight the inevitable typing errors. The main test of the hand will be very simple. Maximum success will be reflected in an undisturbed night's sleep. Just imagine!!

Thursday February 11th 2010

February 2008:
Fortunately another good day has been recorded.

February 2009:
The month of February must suit Peter, as the journal records another peaceful day.

February 2010:
Maximum success has definitely been the order of the night. I cannot remember the last time I slept until ten minutes past eight. There was one little break in the night when I took Peter to the toilet but then I went straight back to sleep. The surgeon has most certainly performed a miracle on my right hand, so I am fully expecting a return to complete control and normality - as far as the hand is concerned - within the next few months. Initial signs are very encouraging. The pharmacist from the Windmill Lane Pharmacy has been most kind in finding, and then delivering, appropriate dressings for me to use, once I can start to change the current dressing.

Friday February 12th 2010

February 2008:
A day of patient excellence has been recorded.

February 2009:
Again an excellent day has been recorded with particular reference to the way Peter coped with - or even ignored - the presence of the children. It is good to look back and to be reminded that we have had some very good days and Alzheimer's has not always scored all the points!!!

February 2010:

Lillian, a close family friend, visited today - after a long absence due to her many cat-minding duties in and around the North West. Joe and Amber came after school, before getting ready to leave for Joe's birthday celebration in Ripon. A good dinner was had by all!! Peter has been in good order and spent a long time organising the cleaning materials in the kitchen and utility room. The hand is doing very well and I have been able to use it to do almost all jobs with reasonable levels of success and competence. It will be interesting to see how long it takes for the present level of 'pins and needles' to disappear. I do remember that the condition lasted for many months with the broken right arm, but I have to say that, in comparison with the last few weeks, the current level is not unacceptable. If necessary I could learn to live with it - but I shall hope that it is not necessary. I can now play a three note chord with reasonable clarity and I regard this as a very clear sign of good progress. The car is looking very inviting in the drive, but I shall have to resist its blandishments until a few more days have passed. Perhaps I can 'try my hand' next Thursday.

Saturday February 13th 2010

February 2008:

I have commented on some changes which have taken place in Peter but am not quite able to quantify or even accurately describe them. Rachel has summed it up rather more successfully when she writes,

"A few more lights have gone out."

February 2009:
Paul and Muna came to collect Danny and Alex. Peter, amidst all this excitement, spent a calm, silent, peaceful but slightly confused day. He was very puzzled by the sight of the dining table set for six people. Sadly it would not be a puzzle for long!

February 2010:
The hand is responding very well indeed. I changed the first dressing this morning and found everything in excellent order. The embroidery appears to be of a high standard. It will be unpicked next Friday. Rachel, Stephen, Joe and Amber have all gone off to Ripon to celebrate Joe's eighteenth birthday, so Denton is very quiet. I am not too keen on the 'no driving' element of the recovery, but I do feel that once the requisite number of days have passed then I shall be back in good running - or even driving - order. Peter has now noticed the bandage on the hand and is very keen to move it round in circles - the hand I mean, not the bandage. I am slightly less keen but at least he has spotted something different in the environment. He has now developed a great interest in spreading the contents of his book box - the containable one by the chair - over the space surrounding his chair. Should he reach the hallway there could be a need for intervention as he will collide with the toy boxes.

Sunday February 14th 2010

February 2008:
Peter had been very disoriented, and unable to make sense of the process of having a bath and getting into bed. I had taken the four children to The Blue Planet and Rachel had been on call for the morning and part of the afternoon. She reported that Peter had been more tottery than usual.

February 2009:
Peter was reported as being calm, silent and seemingly contented. On reflection it seems reasonable to note that, increasingly, silence has begun to be a regular feature of Peter's life. I have no reason to suppose that any significant frustration is part of the silence. He does not seem to be agitated, which I might expect if I thought he was struggling to find a way of communicating what he is feeling. I have already mentioned that I suspect Peter's brain has stopped trying to communicate very much - in any way. What we cannot know is whether the brain has stopped trying to communicate because the means no longer exist, or whether it has nothing to communicate. I suspect the latter, but can find no plausible evidence to support my suspicions. The calm day has included many opportunities for folding, straightening, sorting and lining up, not forgetting a determined assault on the Lever Arch File. A big plus has been a reduction of puddles, due to a strict adherence to the supervision code which has, in turn, resulted in a reduction in the use of Mr. Muscle Cleaner with added Bleach.

February 2010:
Even though Spring is just around the corner - or at least within hailing distance of next month - Peter has been increasingly reluctant to get up. Had we been recording the rising time, then such times would, more often than not, have been after three o'clock. Once up he spends a little time reorganising the washing-up bowl, dish cloth and tea towel before withdrawing to the Study, eating an apple, drinking half a cup of coffee and then falling asleep. A new occupation in the evening is to investigate the fit of the carpet in the hall - particularly the part under the radiator. The carpet was fitted, extremely well, in 1996 and does not present any visible problems. However, Peter seems to take pleasure kneeling on the floor, smoothing out invisible wrinkles, picking up and pocketing sometimes visible fluff, before grasping the radiator and pulling himself to his feet. It is then time to have another sleep. My plan to start bedtime before midnight has met with little success because I keep falling asleep in the chair. Perhaps that insidious disease, known as sleeping sickness, has gained a foothold in the house!! Better luck from now on. The hand continues to improve and is feeling much more comfortable.

Monday February 15th 2010

February 2008:
Again the problem of understanding the sequences and processes involved in matters such as dressing have presented one or two problems.

February 2009:

The day has followed the recent trend of being shorter - due to a later rising time - very quiet and not very active. Sorting and folding seem to have been reduced, with an increase in the number of lapses into sleep. Molly and William will be coming tomorrow and staying until Wednesday tea-time, so it will be interesting to see if Peter notices their presence in the house.

February 2010:

A calm, silent and contented day has been reported with its fair share of sorting, folding, Lever Arch File massacring, plus, provided the strict routine is followed, a reduction in puddles and a subsequent saving on the use of Mr. Muscle with added Bleach.

Tuesday February 16th 2010

February 2008:

The children's holiday and the abundance of Playmobil and Fisher Price toys have combined to puzzle, challenge, but also stimulate Peter's somewhat reduced understanding of changes on the domestic front. I have reported seeing a level of satisfaction in the lining up and arranging of the toys, coupled with a certain style in the presentation of the final parade - or line up. The days of the children's holiday have been wonderful days.

February 2009:
Although Peter was unable to cope with dressing himself he managed to make the bed before lunchtime. This has been an excellent achievement and one we should acknowledge.

February 2010:
Molly and William arrived this morning for their two days holiday and so the day got off to a very good beginning. I am still trying to work out what has changed in Peter's condition. That is a somewhat foolish description of whatever is left of his brain. We all know what the word condition is supposed to mean but I am still left baffled by some of the things he cannot do. Today's consoling action has been a great concentration on straightening the already perfectly tailored chair upholstery. Molly and William have brought their own brand of sparkle and delight into the home and the sight of them, sleeping so happily in their beds, is a consolation prize beyond price.

Wednesday February 17th 2010

February 2008:
I took Danny and Alex to Keele to meet Paul and so bring a lovely few days to an end. Rachel found Peter reluctant to get up and not too willing to be helped with the dressing. He seemed to be very muddled.

February 2009:
With my brain in its present poor state I find myself wondering if I actually wrote the entry for 2009. A thought

process was triggered by a few comments from John Suchet - Hercule Poirot's (aka David Suchet's) brother - on the subject of his wife's diagnosis with Alzheimer's disease. For him it was shocking and distressing that she had no knowledge of her condition and so they could not discuss it. This shows exactly how very different we are in the coping strategies we use. For me there is great consolation in knowing that Peter is totally unaware of his condition. We had never actually moved beyond the furious and outraged acceptance of memory loss.

February 2010:
We have had a wonderful day today with Molly and William. Joe and Amber spent the morning in Manchester with Lillian - celebrating her birthday - and joined us in the mid-afternoon. Peter has been very happy today. Perhaps the effect of the children in the house is beginning to creep into his existence. What a wonderful thing that would be!! I do not think his muscle tone is too impressive these days. Not if his walking is supposed to be any measure of tone. There has been a most definite deterioration in his mobility. I did note last night that climbing up the stairs is rather more demanding of both time and energy. The extra rail is, as one would hope, a real friend in time of need and Peter seems to appreciate its presence. Certainly he felt moved to grip the section at the top of the stairs and shake it vigorously. Without first-hand knowledge of his muscle-tone I would have felt that the rail was under threat. Mark's friend - Mark the Gasman - cometh tomorrow to fit a new control panel

for the boiler, so that I do not have to crouch down with a large torch in order to find out exactly what is going on - or even off. The hand wound is looking very healthy. Some stitching has split but what could one expect with dementia, half-term and the family genes. Amber's best Girl Guide First Aid dressing was very good indeed and needed no adjustment - unlike mine!! I am going to see if I can take the car out tomorrow. If I put the splint on top of the dressing then the palm of the hand will be very well protected and it could mean that I can drive over to the Alexandra on Friday for the sutures to be removed. Molly and William have gone home - which is my penance for Ash Wednesday!

Thursday February 18 2010

February 2008:
I wrote a lot on this day two years ago, much of which is very relevant in 2010, but I think it would be a good idea to leave the day with the wonderful statement Danny made - after spending nine days at my address. To quote Danny,

> "Grandma, I don't think there is really anything the matter with Grandad. He smiles and is polite. He remembers his manners and can eat his food nicely. He looks kind and I like this Grandad."

It would be wonderful to think that the same opinion would be expressed today.

February 2009:

Today's experiment was to see the effect of leaving Classic FM on, at a low level, during the time Peter spent in the Study. I would say now, after one year, that the experiment worked, from my point of view, but I am not convinced that Mozart and Bach were engaging with Peter. Dynamics do present a little problem but, more frequently, there is anxiety over the source of the sound. Perhaps the questioning of source indicates a slightly more sophisticated mental process than would seem likely??

February 2010:

I can only comment on a day of exceptional calm and quiet. Joe and Amber were here for much of the day but even they were quiet and calm. My calm and quiet demeanour was influenced, on several occasions, by my decision to drive over to the Alexandra to have the stitches removed. This decision is causing me a great deal of anticipation and excitement. Debi, the Psychiatric nurse, will visit in the morning so I shall discuss the quiet state of Peter's existence, and see how it fits in with supposedly normal trends.

A glance at these comparisons is not revealing very much in the way of new and exciting information. I am becoming increasingly aware of the somewhat static nature of the disease at this moment, and am wondering exactly what I am going to make of this study. However, the search goes on, in the expectation that something, surely, will be revealed. Perhaps, if you are at a similar stage in the caring situation, you too will have been struck by the tedium which seems to be an ingredient of this disease. If so, it may be that you are successfully creating some mild excitement for yourself, as one of your coping strategies. I do hope so.

Chapter Two - We have the questions but very few answers

Friday February 19th 2010

February 2008:
This day has gone on record as an outstanding day with Peter being in excellent order and doing his best.

February 2009:
Unlike last year, today has seen a very obvious link between aggression and not understanding the requirements of the world in which Peter has found himself. Again it really comes down to the whole business of management. When managed correctly Peter can be calm. When there is a blip in the system he is very quickly thrown into confusion and a state of apprehension, or possibly fear of what has become the unknown. Sufficient to say that we can see levels of aggression which we would be well advised to reduce or, preferably, avoid altogether. There is little future for any of us here if the aggression is not contained. I am absolutely certain that it can be contained. This is an example of the genie needing to stay in its bottle - the genie being aggression, of course, not Peter.

February 2010:
The sutures have been removed from my hand and I am ready to pick up the lightweight cudgels I put down ten days ago. I am very happy with the outcome and look forward to seeing an increase in dexterity, grip and control. As I mentioned yesterday I did ask Debi whether or not Peter's current state of calm was a normal development in the Alzheimer cycle. Debi seemed to think that it was not part and parcel of the condition. She favours the idea that, somehow or other, we have created an environment and routine in which Peter can be calm and peaceful. She also felt that, in any other situation, it would take a very short time for aggression to be shown and for his behaviour to change - for the worse. If this is, indeed, the way things are working then extraordinary tedium seems a very small price to pay for calm, and that highly desirable commodity known as the Quiet Life. As one who is keen on the Quiet Life - it does, after all, open up all sorts of different possibilities - I hope we will all jog along, as we are, and do what we can to maintain the status quo - including Peter.

There is not a great deal to mention these days but it may be that February will go on record as a quiet month in our home. There is one thing to mention. Two days ago I found Peter standing by the sink and sucking at the cuff of his jacket. The jacket is now elderly and part of the cuff, which had previously been bound with black binding, had frayed slightly revealing those white threads one often sees in worn black cloth. Peter had been cleaning his teeth only five minutes earlier and I rather suspect that he thought the white threads might have been flecks of toothpaste. Perhaps he thought the best way to remove toothpaste from his jacket would be by licking it off. If this is what he had in his mind then it again suggests a level of mental activity which may not be reflected in other less exciting situations. He was happy enough for me to change the offending jacket for his other jacket. This is a new level of excitement which deserves documentation.

Saturday February 20th 2010

February 2008:
Another very good day, with Rachel mentioning that Peter had tried to discuss something connected with height but, although the discussion was animated and hand gestures were in evidence, she was not able to make any sense of what was going on. This does not appear to upset Peter.

February 2009:
Peter had been very tired today but not too tired to organise the kitchen. Today he had sorted items into separate groups according to some obvious attributes. Any nursery or infant teacher would have been very encouraged to see the practical application of this sorting and grouping concept. This activity is set to become an important part of Peter's work programme.

February 2010:
If I say that today has been another February day I shall not be referring to the weather, but rather to Peter's very quiet and peaceful reaction to the day. All in all today has been immensely enjoyable and very productive.

Sunday February 21st 2010

February 2008:
I noted, with interest, that Peter definitely appears to be less and less aware of his surroundings and certainly less aware of what, or even who, is going on.

February 2009:
A most excellent day has been reported - for which many thanks.

February 2010:
I shall have to say, 'Another February day,' by which, of course, I mean that Peter has been cool (nothing to do with today's snowfall), calm and collected. Two days ago I noticed an odd little mark on the side of Peter's left big toe. The mark puzzles me because I cannot see that it is the result of pressure from his shoe and it does not seem to be the result of a knock. I shall watch and note its progress. Having written about its existence will probably ensure its total disappearance by the end of the week!

Monday February 22ⁿᵈ 2010

February 2008:
This is the first record of Peter interfering with whatever I was doing or preparing in the kitchen. Not content with lining up all available crockery and cutlery, he also needed to line up and organise every item I had in my hands.

February 2009:
A reluctance to get up and face the world has been reported. Once up, he coped valiantly.

February 2010:
Following the expected custom for the month of February, Peter has enjoyed a calm peaceful day. I wonder if the folding and sorting he practises reflects therapy or habit. I would like to think there was some benefit from all that work he does each day.

Tuesday February 23ʳᵈ 2010

February 2008:
Another good day has been recorded.

February 2009:
The nature of the attacks on the Lever Arch File has been carefully analysed. The whole problem lies in the fact that Peter wishes to straighten the arch manually - rather in the manner of a ring binder. I fear there is no way round this problem.

February 2010:
Today has been the usual quiet February day we have come to expect. There was, however, one slight difference. I returned from choir practice to find Peter sitting on the bean bag nearest to the TV in the music room. This has not happened before, as far as I am aware. He had obviously been straightening the kitchen and must have decided that he needed to sit down. This is a definite change in behaviour. I wonder what we can expect from tomorrow. Possibly absolutely anything . . . or even nothing! Another question of 'Watch this space.'

Wednesday February 24th 2010

February 2008:
There has been mention of tedium associated with the daily routine. We must be deeply immersed in both routine and tedium as it would seem that very little has changed in two years - except that we are greatly skilled in handling both those commodities.

February 2009:
If I say 'more of the same' I am sure you will understand exactly what I mean. Tranquility reigns supreme.

February 2010:
Amber has worked most carefully and persistently in pasting down some of those pieces of wallpaper which love to pop out when no-one is looking. She is already demonstrating good wallpapering skills . . . and will soon

be taking orders. Peter has not been affected by her attention to the work he carried out nearly sixteen years ago. I have to say that the wallpaper is really in need of replacement but I cannot quite see how that can be achieved at present. Peter has enjoyed another non-challenging, peaceful, satisfying - I hope - and restful February day. Over to you, Rachel, as choir practice calls.

> "For the first time in many months Dad was keen to follow me round for the first half an hour, at one point trying to line me up alongside the table. I resisted and put myself out of view. He then settled for the evening."

Thursday February 25th 2010

February 2008:
It reads, 'not an outstanding day.' Yet it was still a February day!!

February 2009:
There is a useful and interesting point which seems to support the concept of constant supervision being coupled with trying to make life as uncomplicated as possible for Peter. Seemingly this is an attempt to secure the positive rewards of the Simple Life.

February 2010:
Peter is doing a great deal of resting and sleeping but still seems content with his lot. I am certainly very content with the astonishing reduction in pain in my right hand, following the carpal tunnel surgery. It is wonderful to be able to go to sleep and be certain that the only disturbance in the night will be that of taking Peter to the toilet - from time to time. What I have noticed is that he is having a real struggle getting out of bed. Even sitting up is a challenge. I am helping him to find his way to the toilet, but I am leaving him to struggle as he tries, first of all, to sit up then to stand up and then to balance himself before tottering on his way. I am in two minds as to what is the right thing to do but, nevertheless, my instinct is to try and let him manage this vital pattern of events independently, even if it takes a long time. . . Time will tell.

Friday February 26th 2010

February 2008:
Peace and quiet. These words have been very important during the month of February and I note that the quietness of the situation in 2008 prompted a thought about a possible change in direction of the Project.

February 2009:
February is calling the tune again but there has also been a marked increase in the volume of sorting and folding.

February 2010:
Today has been a very busy day with a great number of errands and visits having been required. Peter, however, has continued to be calm and placid. I collected Rosemary this evening and brought her home so that she could cut Peter's hair - and mine. She is extremely good, not only at cutting hair, but in making it possible for Peter to sit quietly, shrouded in green nylon and waiting patiently for the whole operation to come to an end. The end result also looks very good. Bedtime would have been earlier if only I had not fallen asleep again.

Saturday February 27th 2010

February 2008:
There has been a frenzy of folding and lining up, resulting in a satisfying and rewarding day.

February 2009:
There was an interesting report which mentioned that, for the first time, Peter has busied himself moving things from the utility room into the kitchen - and vice versa - before lining them up and ordering them according to secret criteria. This movement from A to B is a new development and may need to be watched!!!

February 2010:
We have enjoyed an outstandingly successful day today. There was an interesting lesson to be learnt by the Management Team this morning. The upstairs toilet door

was closed when Peter got out of bed and made his way across the landing. The sight of a closed door caused him some consternation as he must have realised that something was different. The doors of both the upstairs and downstairs toilet are always open, thus making the toilet itself very visible. What Peter did this morning was interesting. He turned away from the closed door and made his way back to the bedroom. I quickly led him back to the toilet lest matters deteriorate. It was very confusing and Peter's brain struggled to make him understand what was required of him. The object of the lesson is that every effort needs to be made to keep the routine in place and not allow barriers of any nature to appear. For this reason I have decided against my brainwave of having all the rooms re-papered. Peter's routes from here to there - and back again - would be severely compromised.

Sunday February 28th 2010

February 2008:
The month of February ended on a high as far as calm was concerned.

February 2009:
Again we could not have asked for a happier conclusion to the month of February - as far as Alzheimer's is concerned, of course. Sorting and folding have taken on a whole new identity and, with hindsight, I can see the development of a major form of therapy.

February 2010:

Although it was rather late before Peter felt able to allow himself to get up (by late I mean well after half past three in the afternoon), he has maintained the standard he set for the month of February. Sleep has occupied at least half of the waking hours - yes, that is exactly what I mean - but those lovely words, peace, calm and apparent contentment are all very appropriate. Perhaps I shall decide to continue with peace, calm and contentment for a little longer. At the moment I feel there is more I could be looking for, or working out, or even understanding, but it will definitely need a clear investigation or, which would be much more welcome, a flash of inspiration. So, for the time being, 'Welcome tomorrow' and whatever it brings - including the March Hare.

Monday March 1st 2010

March 2008:

Today's main focus has been Peter's disorientation and his inability to make much, if any, sense of the spoken word.

I note that it is two years ago today that I removed the functioning part of the front door chain, to prevent Peter from locking me out of the house.

March 2009:

Again there is reference to a further deterioration in Peter's cognitive skills.

March 2010:

There is something worthy of comment today. Having spent two and a half peaceful hours, including sleeping in his chair within thirty minutes of having dressed, Peter came into the kitchen just as I was preparing some dinner for Joe and Amber to eat, before Rachel came to collect Amber and to take her to her climbing lesson. That should have been a straightforward happening but, at the sight of six very small quorn breaded nuggets, Peter must have been reminded that he needed some food. I turned my back to place a dish in the oven only to see, as I stood up, Peter standing by the quorn dish and merrily chewing his way through one breaded nugget. This was Amber's food so I had to try and retrieve it. I failed but Peter seemed well pleased with his trophy. He seemed happy to be escorted back into the Study and into his chair. One problem he thinks he has these days involves sitting down on the chair in the bathroom before getting undressed ready for a bath.

I have mentioned before there is a very real mental as well as physical process involved in seeing a chair and then preparing to sit on it. It seems to be the same old problem of not knowing where to place the bottom on the chair.

Tuesday March 2nd 2010

March 2008:
Calmness and confusion have been the order of this rather short day.

March 2009:
Foolishness has been the order of this particular day.

March 2010:
Peter has smiled a great many times today - which has been pleasant. He took it upon himself to dry up two cups and a spoon and then place them carefully on the draining board. It is a long time since he felt able to do this. Negotiating a sitting position is becoming increasingly difficult, but the day has been good.

Wednesday March 3rd 2010

March 2008:
There has been a positive comment on Peter's nimbleness and generally high level of what would seem to be co-operation.

March 2009:
This year I have focused on Peter's increasingly poor balance. He has been so wobbly that I have decided that he must make much more use of the chair in the bathroom when trying to get ready for a bath. This practice has continued over the last twelve months - and life is much easier.

March 2010:
Although Peter had obviously been out of his bed during the morning, by half past two he had still not attempted to eat his breakfast. He was happy to allow his clothes to be put

on and has continued in a happy and peaceful manner throughout the day. He did become very animated when he found Joe and Amber making truffles in the kitchen. It must have looked like food because he started to become very interested in the mixture and, when he saw Joe and Amber licking their spoons, he must have thought they were eating what was rightfully his!! I tried to coax him into the Study with a cup of coffee and two digestive biscuits. He would not be coaxed! Eventually his dinner was hot enough to eat and he decided it looked more inviting than massaged truffles. This is your space, Rachel.

> "I was met with a hard stare but, after surveying my coat, Dad concluded that I was staying and tottered back. He does have a most shuffling gait now."

Thursday March 4th 2010

March 2008:
Peter found putting on his clothes so difficult that, having donned his vest and shirt, he returned to bed until four o'clock. Sequencing is now a serious challenge.

March 2009:
To quote: 'A day of insignificant achievements. On whose part, I wonder! The kitchen was straightened, which should rank as an achievement.' The quote tells us something about the Staff.

March 2010:

Peter seems to be more and more puzzled by the presence of people in the house - this includes me. He inspected Joe, and then Amber was besieged by numerous hard stares, quizzical looks and, worst of all, a determined attempt to steal the thirty truffles she was trying to dip in melted chocolate. He obviously recognised the truffles as food, possibly even forbidden food, but he did his utmost to claim them as his. I have tried to explain to Amber that her Grandad is really trying to communicate just one idea. That is, 'This is my space. You are in it and I really want it for myself so that I can put things in order.' I do not think that Peter is craving company. What he wants is the knowledge that someone - possibly I am that someone - is in the house, but, preferably, not where he wants to be. This could be anywhere at all, downstairs. It is hard to rationalise this at any age but it must seem very bizarre at thirteen years of age. Amber conceals her thoughts so well that it is not entirely easy to decide whether this makes sense to her, or she suspects it is simply some behaviour designed to annoy her. The truffles are very good indeed, so there is no surprise in Peter thinking that he should claim ownership. . .

Friday March 5th 2010

March 2008:
Sequencing is the main problem at present.

March 2009:
Again I am querying how much Peter is able to understand where and how people fit into his life.

March 2010:
Rachel has diagnosed a clear case of sundowning in Peter. I wonder..? Certainly he is particularly active in and around the kitchen when Joe and Amber are here. They must find it somewhat disconcerting to be stared at whenever they are sitting down quietly, minding their own business and trying to watch Agatha Christie's *The Murder of Roger Ackroyd*. Having scrutinized them most carefully he came in the kitchen to advise me on ... well, anything at all, really. He certainly is able to recognise food on a plate and, understandably, is anxious not to miss anything that might be his by right. Three trays present a puzzle which is almost as big as three places at the table. I am wondering whether the new behaviour has anything to do with the longer days. Perhaps he is anxious for more exercise in order to increase his muscle tone. One thing is obvious though: all this scrutinizing, observing and witnessing is making him very tired. After twenty minutes in the kitchen he has to sit down and rest for at least half an hour. The next odd thing is the way he is trying to avoid swallowing his tablets. There is a certain lack of subtlety in the way he takes them from the spoon, appears to swallow, accepts a glass of water to facilitate swallowing and then again appears to swallow. Should I be so naive as to leave the room and collect his food for him I could well come back to find all the tablets,

carefully arranged in a tidy and orderly row, on the small wicker table and so we would need to start all over again. Lillian visited today - which was another puzzle for Peter, which he indicates by shrugging his shoulders. What that means is anyone's guess.

Saturday March 6th 2010

March 2008:
The day was so good that I have claimed to be a perfectly normal person leading a perfectly normal life!!

March 2009:
Debi, the Community Psychiatric Nurse visited today and acquainted herself with the month's activities - or lack of them. She accepts all this with her usual good humour. She has, with her cheerful and supportive personality, been a great source of strength over these many months.

March 2010:
William has been here since lunchtime for his long awaited sleep-over and we are greatly enjoying ourselves. Peter has inspected him closely, smiled at him in a kindly fashion and been very, very busy today. It is better not to stay in any one place for any length of time because Peter will, most definitely, try some sort of moving-on trick. Problem-solving is still evident. Today his razor stopped functioning when he had almost finished shaving. Not to be outdone Peter put the razor down, in a mildly contemptuous manner,

picked up a large red comb and started to comb his clean-shaven upper lip.

Sunday March 7th 2010

March 2008:
One factor becomes increasingly obvious concerning the whole subject of Alzheimer's disease, and that is in the statement:

> "There seems to be little available information on this or any other form of dementia."

Such a statement would not be true two years later. Now there is more factual information on the physical processes involved in the development of this type of dementia. But it would be fair to question the extent to which increased information has effectively improved the understanding and care of people thus afflicted.

March 2009:
Debi visited and, unlike on her previous visits, was actually able to see Peter in the flesh and so see for herself how healthy he looks. A true and honest assessment of muscle tone would have been impossible for all but the truly creative. Nevertheless his appearance and amiable demeanour were both beyond any reasonable reproach.

March 2010:

William and I have greatly enjoyed his sleep-over. He actually slept from 8pm until 8.50am - making, as you will see, a total of twelve hours and fifty minutes. He seemed to feel greatly refreshed. I am more and more certain that the undeniable change in Peter's behaviour may well be due to a basic, even primitive, response to the lengthening day and the warmer weather. It is almost as though he has come out of hibernation, or, at the very least, a period of dormancy. I am not absolutely certain that I am welcoming the change as it seems to be impinging on the way I am conducting the two lives - and it interferes, physically, with the cooking of food.

Monday March 8th 2010

March 2008:

I am still questioning exactly what it is we are trying to understand about how dementia works, but Peter appears to be unconcerned.

March 2009:

A good day has been recorded - so something has been understood by someone.

March 2010:

The inspection of many items of culinary interest has continued for a good hour this evening, otherwise it has been a quiet and calm day. I am not so certain about the contentment because sometimes I felt an element of containment rather than contentment! But perhaps that was on my part.

Tuesday March 9th 2010

March 2008:
There is an increasing level of puzzlement with regard to dressing activities but not enough to cause Peter any concern.

March 2009:
Co-operation versus comprehension. The beginning of the Great Debate.

March 2010:
I am sure the lighter evenings have something to do with Peter's increased level of activity. Perhaps the Spring will ease his situation.

Wednesday March 10th 2010

March 2008:
More problems with the light bulbs so further removals are indicated.

March 2009:
The Management Staff must learn about the results of failure to comprehend - on both sides of the Great Debate

March 2010:
There has been slightly less activity so far but Peter has been very amiable today. It is choir practice tonight so it is over to you, Rachel, and Thank You very much indeed. You will be in charge of all activities.

"Dad has kept his eyes firmly closed all evening, but opened one eye when coffee was delivered. He has balanced the place mat on top of the Lever Arch File with great precision."

Thursday March 11th 2010

March 2008:
A good quiet day, by all accounts.

March 2009:
A year later sees yet another good quiet day.

March 2010:
Today has, to use an odd phrase, beggared belief. I am not sure it should have even started. But it did. Having put a quart's worth of work into the proverbial pint pot I decided to get Peter up and dressed by two o'clock, well before Joe and Amber arrived back from School. Everything appeared to be in good order: toileting, putting on the vest, shirt, tie and jersey and preparing for the underpants. Please note, at this point, that a cunning little dodge is being practised with the shirt. I have, quite deliberately, bought generously cut shirts, with a sixteen inch collar, so the cuffs are also

generous. So generous that, after all this time, it has occurred to me that it may not be necessary to unfasten them at the end of each day before putting the shirt out to wash. This would then mean that tomorrow's shirt would slip over the wrist and so save on time and wear on the fingers - my fingers. It is a masterpiece of erudition, and it works!! But, to revert to the dressing, Peter took exception to something, became very aggressive and refused to be parted from his pyjama trousers. I lost interest and, on hearing Joe return from College, closed the bedroom door - leaving the rest of the clothes on the bed - and went downstairs.

Half an hour later I went upstairs to find Peter dressed and ready to face the world. He had retrieved the pyjama jacket and put it on over his vest, shirt and jersey. He was wearing his long johns and I could see a smart blue trim at the top of the pants, which suggested that he was still wearing his pyjama trousers under his long johns. He was wearing his shoes and socks - with the laces fastened on his shoes. He was also trying to pull the bed into some sort of shape. I managed to put his trousers on and then take off the pyjama jacket. Sartorial elegance had been severely compromised by the jacket. His suit jacket looked much smarter. He managed to come downstairs and clean his teeth. I gave him his electric razor and he started to clean his teeth again. The vibration did not appear to affect him but I felt I had to stop the fun. The day continued with the time being fairly evenly split between folding and sleeping. As he was asleep at seven o'clock it seemed reasonable to fit in a call I had not managed to make this morning. I was back home just before nine o'clock. Peter was still asleep but there were definite signs of activity in the kitchen. At half past ten I gave Peter his tablets and he had a mouthful of tepid coffee. At half past eleven I decided to bring the day to an end. Everything seemed to be calm and peaceful until, having raised the chair to the correct height, I put out my hand to help Peter to stand up. All movements had been as usual. I was not aware of any hurried or jerky movements on my part, but, something was not right. Peter suddenly stiffened in the chair, so that he could not be moved out and became very aggressive again. He not only looked aggressive but he clenched his fists and tried to punch the air - all accompanied by angry vocals. By this stage it seemed incredibly dull and tedious so I turned out the Study light and went upstairs, where the bath was filling with very tempting looking bubbly water. I undressed and got straight into the bath. What bliss. Having decided on a definite, possibly murderous, course of action, which is probably better left unwritten, I then decided to give him another chance. Second time round was trouble free and straightforward. Taking off all three layers of clothing - remember the extra pyjama trousers - was rather more of a struggle than usual and Peter played his new trick of pretending that his feet have been fastened to the floor and cannot be moved. Pressing the top of the foot will often cause a reflex action which causes the foot to move just long enough to allow Staff to remove the clothing. I also discovered that Peter was wearing my watch on his left wrist. I have been looking for the watch for several days - as well as the nail scissors - so I was happy to retrieve it and impressed by the fact that Peter had fastened the watch round his own wrist - without reference to anybody. The scissors could well turn up before too long. Everything was plain sailing from then on.

Friday March 12th 2010

March 2008:
I read, with horror, about the getting up in the night in order to turn on the bedroom light and to try and empty the contents of the chest of drawers in order to line things up. Removing light bulbs has been a most excellent plan of action.

March 2009:
It was obviously important to report a complete absence of sorting and folding on Peter's part. As for the Lever Arch File, its head is looming again.

March 2010:
I can only report that Peter has had a good day after a rather late start, but I am hoping to end the day before midnight as I am going to Birmingham in the morning.

Sunday March 14th 2010

March 2008:
Sorting, folding and peace . . .

March 2009:
The Lever Arch is reigning supreme.

March 2010:
Today has been a lovely day during which I have celebrated my birthday and the children have celebrated Mothering Sunday. I have received flowers, chocolates and cards to ensure that the day was truly wonderful. Peter has been calm today so I shall close on that note of peace and tranquility.

Monday March 15th 2010

March 2008:
Folding, sorting and reorganising the kitchen have been essential ingredients in the day's programme.

March 2009:
There has been further evidence of the confusion Peter experiences when anyone else is in the house. He has been doing his best to be helpful - particularly when I am in the kitchen.

March 2010:
Today could have been a very testing time indeed. Peter was up by half past two, by which time both Paul and Lillian had arrived. Within the next half hour Rachel had arrived, Paul and Rachel had gone and Amber had arrived. At six o'clock Rachel and Joe returned and then left with Amber. At half past seven both Lillian and I left. Now, where did that leave us. Peter seemed happy to keep seeing different people at

different times. Each time appears to be the first time - as we know. He was only seriously challenged when he saw plates of dinner for Amber and Lillian. His own was coming within seconds but he was deeply puzzled by the plates and very concerned when they were placed in front of other people. When his own dinner was ready and on the tray he then decided to try and straighten up the chair in the Study - or, to be more accurate, to straighten up the red protective thin cushion. This evening has been quiet. I took Lillian home and returned to Denton to find a tidy kitchen with several new items on view - which had previously been concealed in cupboards. A strange looking sore area has appeared on the right hand side of Peter's face - high up on the hair-line. I am treating it with Sudocrem and am hoping it is not a rodent ulcer. He is rather more unsteady on his feet but does not appear to be concerned.

Tuesday March 16th 2010

March 2008:
It is most interesting to note how long it has taken to establish the general loss of comprehension.

March 2009:
The loss of comprehension - and subsequent apparent lack of co-operation - has become more and more apparent.

March 2010:
The main achievement of the day actually started on Sunday evening. I woke up to an exceptionally cold house and

quickly discovered that there was no heat in the house. Hot water? Yes. Hot radiators? No. I searched for a possible explanation. I searched for helpful documentation and even rang the Gas Man - Mark's friend. He advised me and I followed his helpful advice but I did not achieve any heat at all. I went into the hall to collect my bag and, for some unknown reason, I stopped by the small thermostat next to the mirror. Miraculously I noted that it looked different from usual and, once the brain had lurched into action, I realised that the device had been switched off - by person or persons unknown!! I have concluded that the thermostat was showing a pointer which was not at right angles to the base and this would have caused Peter some concern - if not offence. Once I had reset the thermostat we had heat and good humour on the part of the Management Team. After a very good day and quiet evening there was a slight change. The first incident was the spillage of a large cup of black coffee over the Study carpet. Peter had swallowed his tablets with one mouthful of coffee before putting the cup down on the table. The problem was that he let go of the cup before his hand was anywhere near the coffee table. Hence the spillage. An immediate and vigorous cleaning operation has not yet succeeded in removing the stain. Rachel assures me that it will eventually go way - given plenty of treatment. That could be true of most of us. We too could go away - given enough treatment!!

Wednesday March 17th 2010

March 2008:
Seemingly I have achieved everything I set out to achieve. What a worthy comment. It makes me feel very proud - two years on.

March 2009:
A very good day, but Peter shows no sign of knowing whether or not I am in the house. Perhaps this is a mixed blessing - for some of us.

March 2010:
This morning's wet floor was due to my failure to wake up when Peter got out of bed. But I am still trying to work out how dry pyjamas match up with this wet floor. Peter slept for a long time today but seemed very willing to get up and be dressed. I hope, Rachel, that you have a quiet evening. Peter has spent a long time scrutinising different activities involving Joe and Amber. He was particularly interested in the making and dipping of rum truffles - which have been hidden in the fridge, Rachel. You and Peter are more than welcome to have one truffle each but do not let Peter see where they are as that could be the one thing he remembers today!!!!!

There has been no movement at all. In fact he spent most of the evening with his legs stretched out in front of himself and his hands tucked under his legs. I can't say it looked very comfortable.

Thank you, Rachel for enabling choir practice to take place!

> "Legs are now supporting the Lever Arch File and his hands are clutching, even embracing, his book on Oliver Cromwell."

Thursday March 18th 2010

March 2008:
Sometimes I am struck by the unconscious truth recorded two years ago:

"It is astonishing how smoothly the day can run if everybody remembers what they are supposed to be doing and can get it all in the right order."

March 2009:
There have been marked signs that the worm is thinking of turning. I am glad to say that, by the end of the day, the worm had thought better of it and had realised that, by spending a lot of time and energy helping Peter to negotiate his way through the day, the day itself was able to end on a positive note.

March 2010:
I have written a lot today but it has disappeared from the screen. I have tried in every way to retrieve the work but have not met with any success. So, here is a very brief synopsis. Peter was late in waking up and when he did eventually surface I noticed his eyes were not focusing. His

eyes were rolling round in the eye sockets. He did, however, rally within ten or twelve seconds and try to sit up. This took some time but was eventually achieved. I sometimes wonder just where Peter's centre of gravity lies. His shape, when walking, does not appear to match the process as he is very tottery and bent. He will then astound me by kneeling down quickly to straighten up a piece of fluff and will then shuffle over to some suitably supportive piece of furniture and stand up with relative ease.

Friday March 19th 2010

March 2008:
Peter spent ninety minutes trying to make a small mirror fit into its outer frame. He was not disturbed by the fact that he could not make it fit - in any way. Rachel was forced to report the theft of her tea - by her own father.

March 2009:
This is interesting because I threatened to cancel the day on account of a disgraceful lapse of suitable and acceptable behaviour.

March 2010:
Debi visited this morning and mentioned, in passing, that she thought the doctor had said that Peter had not only Alzheimer's dementia but also vascular dementia - which I thought rather suggested an element of greed or even one-upmanship. I find myself wondering if Peter has anything going through his mind when he sits in the chair with his

eyes closed. He is not fast asleep all the time. Does he think he feels comfortable in his chair? Does he hope it's dinner time? Does he wonder what is going on? Or has he found the secret of life?

Saturday March 20th 2010

March 2008:
It was Maundy Thursday but Peter was not aware. There was nothing to report this time. All was under control. I wonder whose? History does not tell us.

March 2009:
Joe and Amber came to stay overnight and, as part of the evening's entertainment we went to a performance of *Tiptoe Through The Tulips* - presented by the local amateur dramatic society. It was very good indeed and both Joe and Amber slept well that night. Peter was calm and well rested as he did not choose to get up too early.

March 2010:
Coincidentally, Joe and Amber came round tonight and we went to a performance of *I'll Get My Man* - presented by the same local amateur dramatic society. Sadly for me they were not able to stay overnight but we greatly enjoyed the play and felt that, as a community, we were very lucky to be able to access a performance such as the one we enjoyed tonight. With so many changes within our society, and so many changes in the way we live, it seemed a remarkably lovely old-fashioned thing to be able to go round to the local

Community Centre and see the dramatic society putting on - and so obviously enjoying - this rather dated but still highly entertaining farce. We all loved it and the atmosphere within the centre was very friendly - not unlike the community itself. The day has been good and Peter seemed very content when I returned after the play.

Sunday March 21st 2010

March 2008:
Peter was able to note the arrival of two guinea pigs and one rabbit, as Rachel and family set off for their holiday in Dorset. Holiday pet care is another one of our distractions.

March 2009:
This time Peter responded, very vocally, to the sudden noise caused by his shoe when I allowed it to drop on the bathroom floor. The response was, "Oh! Crash! Bang!!" This must have been somewhat exceptional as it was obviously considered worthy of comment.

March 2010:
Because of Peter's excellent level of helpful co-operation he was out of bed, dressed, shaved, had his breakfast and cleaned his teeth within one hour of my return from church. This was wonderful, because it meant that Joe and I could catch the bus to Stockport in time to see a splendid performance of her poetry by Pam Ayres. We greatly enjoyed the whole two and a half hours - although the adolescent Joe was possibly the only person there who had

yet to celebrate his fiftieth birthday!! He was quite unconcerned. On our return I found that Peter had eaten none of the extra dishes of snacks and interesting biscuits I left in the kitchen for him to find and eat - if hungry. There was no indication that he had realised that he was on his own in the house. He did enjoy his dinner, though, and has spent the entire evening resting quietly and recharging his batteries - for what purpose I know not. Are we still on a plateau, I wonder. I do not think I am making much progress in charting this disease. I am also not convinced about the way one might expect the disease to proceed as it has occurred to me - not for the first time - that most of what one is told is little more than guesswork.

Monday March 22nd 2010

March 2008:
A fair day by all accounts - which means neither good nor bad.

March 2009:
The report suggests a regrettable day which may be best forgotten.

March 2010:
Today has been unbelievably busy but Peter has not been responsible for the extra business. I am still searching for some reasonable answer to the oft repeated question, 'What do we really know about Alzheimer's?' Apart from a few points connected with dead brain cells and a lack of oxygen

to the brain there seems very little to be of much use to either patient or carer in the situation. I will try again tomorrow, when the day may be less fraught.

Tuesday March 23rd 2010

March 2008:
Apart from the arrival of the guinea pigs, Artful and Dodger, and one lop-eared rabbit called Jinx there has been little to challenge Peter. There has been more than a little with which to challenge me. The biggest challenge is trying to hold onto utensils, food, crockery, tins, papers and almost anything one might care to mention - except guinea pigs and a rabbit. The final ranking was 8/10 so there must have been some unrecorded shining moments.

March 2009:
This must be the quote of the week.

> "He has done his best. Too many puddles. Ranking for the day is 2/10."

March 2010:
I am no nearer solving the puzzle presented by Alzheimer's but I am beginning to suspect that the dearth of reportable news may have more to do with Alzheimer's than my lack of creativity. If I consider the narratives as a whole, not extracts taken out of context, I see a much clearer picture of the way Peter had been each day. Nowadays most of the time is spent in sleeping. I do generally regard this as a

blessing and a natural escape from the horror of having lost connection with one's brain.

Wednesday March 24th 2010

March 2008:
Peter obviously impressed me by the way he washed his cereal bowl and spoon - before hiding them in the laundry basket. The day was very good.

March 2009:
I noted with delight a total absence of puddles - which meant the day was good.

March 2010:
If I were trying to write an interesting book about this stage of Alzheimer's disease I would be struggling to find anything to retain the reader's interest. Why should this be? Perhaps it is because, having spent all this time noting what was going on, we have now reached the stage where very little, if anything notable, is actually happening. Perhaps this is a very passive and non-eventful stage. Or, perhaps I have ceased to notice signs which may exist but are scarcely visible. I do think Peter would be happy to stay in bed all day long - were I to allow such a thing. But, on reflection, I did notice something when I was dressing him this afternoon. He suddenly started to engage in responses to non-existent conversations. He seemed to be reciting a litany of useful social comments. I did try to fit my responses into his pattern - but I suspect we both ended up

talking what might be perceived as nonsense. Have you any ideas for discovering the track again, Rachel?

Rachel was quite unable to comment tonight, but she did suggest that she had been required to listen to more sentences than usual, so perhaps there is some intellectual activity or agitation taking place.

Thursday March 25th 2010

March 2008:
Apart from Jinx, the visiting rabbit, having a day of wild behaviour - aided and abetted by William and Molly - the day was an outstanding success. Perhaps Peter realised that he could not hope to compete with Jinx!! But, perhaps more significantly, the TV *Horizon* programme featured a most interesting investigation into aspects of the human mind. Included in the programme was a sequence on Alzheimer's disease. One particular lady, whose husband had been diagnosed with the condition at the age of only fifty-eight, described the disease in the following way.

"When a person has Alzheimer's disease it is as though he or she is dying on the inside out."

Which is so very true. The person may appear to be entirely fit and well and yet be in the process of losing every part of his or her personality and being. The cruelty of the disease knows no limits.

March 2009:
After an exemplary start to the day, Rachel, who was second in command during the evening, reported great agitation and a failure to settle. On my return, soon after ten in the evening and having been singing with the Police Choir near Bolton, I was just in time to witness a distinct fall from grace. This brings us to the subject of inappropriate urination - not so much the How or the Where, rather more the Why.

March 2010:
I am tempted to write, "Well, here's a turn up for the book," - always supposing one should be written. After all, who knows? After the non-events of the last few days, today seems, by comparison, to have been most eventful. On my return at half past twelve, after visiting a friend in Didsbury, I came into the house in time to hear the sound of a spoon scraping against what turned out to be Peter's cereal bowl. When I took him a cup of coffee it became evident that he was very keen to walk around and examine the chest of drawers and the contents. He found one of a pair of gold cuff links - belonging to his father - and arranged the link on the top. He then sat on the bed and, after refusing his coffee, allowed his clothes to be put on. Cleaning his teeth seemed a totally new experience. Shaving was another strange requirement. Peter was then wandering around, lining up the kitchen and sorting the plates. He was busy so I was somewhat concerned when, on leaving, at half past two, to collect the children from school, Peter was still in the kitchen rather than sitting in his chair. When I returned

home it was twenty past four and, to my astonishment, Peter was still wandering about, lining up and sorting out. He had made no attempt to drink his coffee and he continued to be busy until dinnertime. Dinner took a long time to eat and there were two visits to the toilet between five and half past six.

Watch this space for further excitement.

Friday March 26th 2010

March 2008:
Although reluctant to get out of bed until four o'clock, Peter had a busy time in the day when he did a great deal of sorting and reorganising in the kitchen. It is essential to leave the materials readily available for sorting and reorganising. This is Peter's work and has to be treated as such.

March 2009:
This was the first time I started to look for a clear definition of what constitutes incontinence. It should be simple enough to deduce that incontinence - or a failure to be continent - is the result of the brain failing to communicate, successfully, the right message to the bladder, at the appropriate time. But there will also be the situation of receiving the message, but not knowing how to respond. It should, as far as I can see, be easy to define, but the reality is much more complicated.

March 2010:

It is now half past eight in the evening and I have to report that, so far, the last twenty four hours have been puddle-free. I will not jump to the conclusion that there is any substance in the suggestion I offered yesterday - but I live in hope. The day has been quiet and uneventful, and the sorting and lining up has not yet happened. Have we reached another plateau and are we stopping for the duration? We shall only know after the event but I am starting to feel that I must do something constructive with all this material.

If I look back to the entry for November 1st 2007 I see that I have actually put forward a reason for the Project coming into being.

"It is my hope that something constructive will emerge from this Project which will improve Peter's quality of life, and even provide some ideas for helping other families caught in the grip of Alzheimer's disease or any other form of dementia."

After two years and five months I realise that, for very good reason, the quality of life for the person with Alzheimer's is totally dependent on the quality of life of the carer. This is not a selfish observation but it is a realistic observation.

Saturday March 27th 2010

March 2008:
There was an interesting sequence when I was preparing apples for an apple crumble. Peter saw them and decided that each piece of apple needed to be dried on a tea towel. Bizarre it may be but at least there was some logic in the fact that a towel was used to dry something wet.

March 2009:
We appear to have had a puddle-free, stress-free, calm day with Peter being in very good order.

March 2010:
I woke up to find Peter standing by his side of the bed. He then walked over to the chest of drawers. Ever alert, I jumped out of bed and quickly changed his pyjamas. This time there was no protest when I changed the trousers, so that was a big bonus. Once Peter was back in bed I went towards the bathroom to get dressed ready for my drive down to Birmingham.

On my return from Birmingham, Peter had eaten two breakfasts and was considering the emergency plate containing another apple and a digestive biscuit. There have been several tremors today. Two involving only the face and three involving the face and body.

Sunday March 28th 2010

March 2008:
The day was cancelled due to a major blip - too shocking perhaps to record!!

March 2009:
Peter had managed to locate and eat the breakfast I had left by the bed before I set off for Birmingham. He also co-operated with the dressing procedure, so all was well.

March 2010:
This plateau is very flat indeed. I have searched in vain for some indication of originality in behaviour but have found nothing. The idea of changing direction seems very sensible at the moment. The new little dodge of leaving the bathroom door open, and thus allowing a greater circulation of air to speed up the evaporation of condensation seemed to work last night. There is one little drawback - small as drawbacks go - and that is I do have to make sure I wake up before Peter, and can dash out of the bedroom and close the bathroom door before he has a chance to register two rooms - and the potential for creating havoc. I was awake first last night and so the cunning little ruse worked very successfully.

Chapter Three - Problem solving and thinking aloud

Monday March 29th 2010

March 2008:
There has been another episode of aggression - connected with dressing - but we have all rallied, in the absence of an alternative course of action.

March 2009:
Today appears to have passed uneventfully.

March 2010:
I just managed to wake up in time to follow Peter as he tottered towards the bathroom. Consequently - no puddle. Peter had his breakfast and then went again into the bathroom. I, with great joy, seized the opportunity to make the bed and arrange the clean clothes on top of the bedspread, so that the scene was set for dressing. Peter came back looking pleased and, as I thought, ready to fit in with the current plans. I invited him to sit down on the bed - which he did - and I then started to place the vest over his head before undoing the pyjama jacket buttons. This is the routine we have followed for at least two years. Then the face of thunder appeared and the obvious signs of immediate resistance started. Being unwilling to spend more time on a momentarily un-winnable confrontation I suggested that he might like to undo the buttons himself. It

seemed that he would not like anything of the sort. In fact what he did was to pull his vest firmly over his jacket and to spend some time trying to flatten the inevitable bumps and ridges. The jacket sleeves then presented a problem because they were not long enough and neither would they fasten at the wrist. I took the tray down, washed up, measured out the toothpaste, lined up the razor, played the piano - loudly - for half an hour, and then went back upstairs. The jersey was on and the pyjama jacket collar was arranged, around the round neck of the vest and the V-neck of the jersey. The socks were on the feet and pulled carefully over the bottom of the pyjama trouser legs. Peter had the underpants and suit trousers in his hands and was trying to wrap them round his legs. I managed to remove the pyjama trousers without removing the socks and, after a while, managed to put on the underpants - the long john variety. Trousers and shoes followed reasonably enough and I left him with the suit jacket. Peter managed to fit this on but was now severely challenged by the collar and various flaps of the pyjama jacket which had escaped from the confines of the vest. I returned and then searched valiantly for a phrase to describe the general effect. Sartorial Elegance did not spring to mind. In the end I abandoned the attempt and we came downstairs to the toothbrush and razor. I am rather glad I had put the paisley patterned tie in the drawer before Peter wound it round his neck. I went downstairs again. Peter seemed to be taking a long time to come downstairs so I went to investigate. He was bumping himself down the stairs on his bottom. "Ah!" said I. I then heard him say, with the utmost clarity, "Am I being summoned?" There could only be one answer so I said it. "Yes." The rest of the day has been restless with a great deal of time and attention being spent on posting the pyjama jacket collar inside the vest. As the jacket is larger than the vest there has been very little sign of success and even less of elegance - sartorial or otherwise.

Tuesday March 30th 2010

March 2008:
I have noted that Peter is becoming increasingly agitated when I am trying to speak on the phone. There has also been an increase in hand wringing, puffing, panting and sighing. Apart from these distress signals I ranked the day as manageable. Was I right? I can only hope my better judgement had not deserted me.

March 2009:
There has been the first report of a wet bed and wet pyjamas with Peter showing no sign of awareness. I have certain contingency plans in operation which means that damage is limited.

March 2010:
Lillian, Joe, Amber, William and Molly were all here today, which did cause Peter some puzzlement and not a little consternation. He did, however, appear to be coping. There was a good deal of inspection of people and rooms but the real reaction came in the evening. Rachel collected Joe and

Amber at the end of the day and I then took William and Molly to meet Joanna in Bredbury and then, at seven o'clock, I took Lillian back to Eccles. I suspect that Peter had spent most of that time moving things in the kitchen but, when I returned, he decided to line up the chairs and straighten the bean bags. I wonder how much time he had spent in looking for missing bodies. There was a great deal of sign language - in the form of ample gesticulations - but it all proved to be beyond my comprehension. This went on for over two hours. He was then able to settle in the Study and fall asleep. Bath time and the end of the day came and went uneventfully and he seemed glad to get into bed.

Wednesday March 31st 2010

March 2008:
It has come as a relief to me to read that we are managing a somewhat bizarre situation in a reasonably acceptable way and that Peter is enjoying a reasonable quality of life

March 2009:
Manageable puddles are reported together with a serious assault on the Lever Arch File.

March 2010:
Peter seems to be very slightly more connected to the day than he has been for many months. I could almost think that there was some logic in the way he has been moving items from here to there, and he has been trying say some words -

none of which were intelligible to me! I could do a great deal worse than repeat the comment for March 31st 2008.

> "It has come as a relief to me to think that we are managing a somewhat bizarre situation in a reasonably acceptable way and that Peter is enjoying a reasonable quality of life."

This is also an appropriate time to leave any further comparisons and look carefully at the situation we are currently experiencing.

April 1st 2010

This first day of April deserves to stand alone in its achievements while we consider the calm before the . . . unexpected.

Peter is much more tottery on his feet and spends a great deal of his time downstairs resting and/or sleeping in the chair. He seems to be in a calm frame of mind and far from being mindful of the knowledge of his condition. I would also say that Peter is calmer than I have ever known him to be in more than forty-five years. Today would be a high-ranking day, although perhaps I should take into consideration a determined assault on a lavender and chamomile spray air freshener. I have spent several years trying to remove the top of one of these sprays - for perfectly legitimate reasons which now elude me - but I have met with little or no success. Peter, without special training, has managed to achieve what the manufacturers may have hoped was impossible - on Health and Safety grounds. Talent is a wonderful gift.

On a final note I must say that Peter appears to have no difficulty in kneeling down on the floor to straighten up the occasional speck of fluff, or reorganise any book which appears to be out of alignment in the bookcase. He also spends some time in straightening the protective covers on his chair. When I consider how he totters around the house, it is astonishing to see how quickly he can pull himself into a half-standing position and then an almost upright position with minimal support. The absence of comment on puddles means that they are now a normal part of the day and measures have been taken to minimise the inconvenience. These measures are sometimes very successful - and sometimes one wonders why one bothers!!

It is hard to grasp the fact that we have now completed one third of the New Year we celebrated such a seemingly short time ago. These last six hours have taken their toll on Peter's strength so Goodness knows what will have happened to his muscle tone! He is yawning steadfastly so I may have to go and prepare the shower - and so run the risk of being able to get into bed before midnight. So, with that thought firmly in mind, I am going to award the day a gold star and go and heat up the shower room.

Chapter Four - Testing times

Perhaps it would be helpful to look at what Peter can achieve at this particular point in time and see how we all progress from there.

1. Dressing is now almost beyond Peter's capabilities.
2. Appropriate cutlery is essential if he is to feed himself.
3. His speech is generally unintelligible, except for the unexpectedly clear and seemingly irrelevant sentences he utters from time to time. These sentences are often clearly enunciated and encourage me to remember that Peter is still inside his shell. An example of such sentences could be, "No, I am not here," and "I am going there." He still says, "Thank You."
4. He needs to be taken to the toilet as he has difficulty in locating its whereabouts.
5. He no longer objects to tolerating Readibriefs - with built in pads - for use during both the day and the night.
6. He still derives pleasure from looking at his books - particularly at the ground plans of cathedrals and other large buildings. How much he understands, at any given time, is not exactly clear as the ground plans may be held at any angle and will often be upside down. On the other hand, with his architectural skills and knowledge, he may be making sense of the plans without having to read the words.

7. He can still co-operate in the bath/bedtime routine, provided all undressing takes place in the bathroom when the bath is full of water and there are no other distractions - e.g. clothing such as his pyjamas being visible.
8. He can eat his food, using a spoon and fork, provided the food is in a manageable form. By that I mean it needs to be cut up and to fit easily on to the spoon.
9. He is no longer capable of independent walking. This skill was lost on Monday June 1st 2010 when Peter fell out of bed and, although not appearing to have suffered any visible damage, was obviously shaken by the experience. An ambulance was called. Two Paramedics examined him and found his BP normal and an ECG proved to be satisfactory. They helped him downstairs and we waited for the emergency doctor to call. Peter was deemed fit to be at home and the day ended in a normal fashion. The next afternoon I was able to help Peter downstairs and he sat quietly in his chair until the GP arrived and examined him. I had mentioned that Peter seemed to be wincing whenever he tried to move or even when I tried to help him move. I have also noticed a marked increase in what appear to be odd tremors which cause Peter to stiffen, shake and then subside quietly when they have passed. The GP saw Peter having one such tremor.
10. I asked the GP if it would be possible to have Peter assessed by the district nurse team, with a view to being provided with a suitable bed so that I can continue to

look after him at home. I also asked for some advice from the Continence Team. Peter has not been downstairs since he woke up on the morning of Wednesday June 3rd.

Monday June 8th 2010

Today saw the arrival of a team of two district nurses. I took them upstairs and showed them into the bedroom where Peter was sitting, neatly, quietly, passively and uncomprehendingly. He remained sitting neatly, quietly, passively and uncomprehendingly when one district nurse fired her opening shot, "Hallo, Peter. Are you comfortable?" Not understanding the question he was not in a position to formulate an appropriate answer. He merely waved a weak hand, in what was either a gesture of uninvited familiarity, or even an acknowledgement of assent, and gazed, uncomprehendingly, at both ladies. What followed, in the way of conversation, would have been warmly welcomed by any leading pantomime script writer. I shall wait and see if a hospital bed is lurking somewhere on the horizon.

The main object of this particular report is to bring us all up to date with Peter as he is now. Because he is unable to walk without help, Peter is still upstairs. It seems more than likely that I will re-organise our bedroom so that it can become a comfortable 'bed-sit' for Peter. Joe and Amber worked heroically, last week, to help me move the motorised armchair upstairs and into the bedroom. So we have the 'sit' already in place. All we need is the 'bed.' Some of Peter's books are within easy reach, as are the place mat and the Lever Arch File. All essential items are now in place and to hand.

Continence, or lack of it, is the main challenge at present, but I am feeling fairly confident that a reliable way of dealing with the problem will eventually emerge. There is a great deal of trial and error at present, involving a wide range of pads, pants and sheets. We shall, most definitely, overcome.

Saturday June 13th 2010

It is very sobering to realise the very rapid descent we have seen over the last three months and, even more painfully, over the last three weeks. Peter's skills at the end of Stage Two seem to be many and varied although, of course, that is only in comparison with what we have at this moment. Imprisoned in his mind and imprisoned in nappies Peter has taken his place in the reality of the world of dementia. Perhaps there is a reality in that world in the same way as there is a reality in what we might describe as the normal world. I am now inclined to think that Peter is experiencing some level of discomfort when he tries to move. Some of this may be due to stiffness resulting from sitting in one place for too long. It may have something to do with the great effort required in moving his legs and supporting his own weight. It may have something to do with his loss of confidence in moving around. It is, I am sure, very important to keep Peter moving around whenever it is possible otherwise he will, I suspect, become chair-bound and then, very quickly, he will be bed-bound. He seems very content to be upstairs in his chair, looking at his Lever Arch File and making the occasional attempt to squeeze the life out of the File. In that respect nothing changes!! He is still managing to help me to help him in and out of the bath and greatly enjoys the twenty five minutes he spends in the bath each evening. This is not only relaxing for him but also helps undo any damage to his skin, which is, at present, in excellent order. Long may it last. Once we have delivery of the hospital bed I shall start to make one or two changes to the downstairs arrangements, so that a little more space is available.

Sunday June 14th 2010

I am most impressed with the way Peter appears to be able to move himself from A to B when I am invisible, and yet appears unable to take his own weight or move at all when I am visible. My next project will be to design an effective cloak of invisibility for use at strategic moments. Seriously though, Peter's walking is scarcely walking. His gait resembles an upright crouch - if you can imagine such a thing. He is far too nervous to attempt to straighten up - consequently he is tottering whenever he tries to put one reluctant leg in front of the other.

Monday June 15th 2010

I can scarcely believe what has happened this evening. Having spent a quiet, peaceful and not overly productive afternoon and evening sitting in his chair in the bedroom, Peter suddenly decided to drag himself to his feet and make his slow and laborious way to the bathroom, where he spent many minutes spinning the rather loose metal plate covers on the handrails. By the time he was ready to face the world I had run the bath and moved his chair from the side of the bed so that it faced the far wall of the bedroom. This is because, perhaps not surprisingly, the minute Peter sees the chair he is seized by an irresistible urge to sit down in it. This makes getting him into bed an exceedingly difficult slow process - as you will imagine. So, having planned a new route from bath to bed, I now find myself, at eleven o'clock, sitting at the computer while Peter is fast asleep in bed - slightly nearer to his side of the bed than mine, which may mean I have a good chance of staying in bed and not being nudged onto the floor. You may laugh but it has been known to happen. So, how does one celebrate such an eventful turn-around? Do I have a bath and catch an early night or do I play a game of Spider Solitaire? I shall do both and hope that the morning does not come too early!! Eleven o'clock on the same day I welcomed the morning. Such an event has, by and large, only occurred in dreams. Of course, I may be dreaming, but no, I am still awake, so I shall play a quick game of Solitaire and then have a bath.

Chapter Five - Plans to convert a bed-room into a bed-sit

Tuesday 16th June 2010

Half way through the morning another district nurse arrived. She oozed amiability and confidence. I was delighted with the way the discussion went and her approach to Peter. To cut a lovely long story short we are expecting to take delivery of a hospital bed - with padded sides - sometime between nine am and two pm tomorrow. Sadly Peter is not able to share in the anticipation of this event, but he has been very calm and willing to self-help whenever possible. You never know, but Peter's life might just be transformed by the new arrangements.

I have returned from the travesty which rejoiced in the name of the nightly bath. Peter decided that the legs seemingly attached to his body did not belong to him. Consequently he was unable to walk and took the easier option of collapsing in a heap at every opportunity provided on the journey from the bathroom to the bedroom. I have visions of him spending the rest of his life in the hospital bed, with the cot-sides permanently in place and enjoying the life of one of Charlie Bucket's Grandfathers - *Charlie and the Chocolate Factory* by Roald Dahl. He is now in bed, totally exhausted and trying his best to get to the very middle of the bed.

Wednesday June 17th 2010

As if to order, Peter woke up at six o'clock so I was able to get him up and dress him before taking him downstairs. I did not think he would be of great assistance when the time came for the great bedroom makeover. It turned out to be a most convenient and successful spot of organisation and he was able to sleep in the Study through all the excitement of bed-building and wardrobe-shuffling.

At one minute past nine Mark's two friends arrived to move the wardrobes and chest of drawers, in order that a space might be created to receive the eagerly awaited hospital bed. At exactly five minutes past nine two bed-makers arrived, complete with a flat-pack bed. The next ten minutes saw an extremely efficient example of four men organising their own space in order to carry out their own designated work. By ten o'clock the drama was over and I was left with a bed, a remote control, a splendid cushion pad for Peter's mechanised chair and two very slippery sheets to help in moving Peter from one awkward position to another - in bed of course. By mid-day everything was in its rightful place and some sort of order had been created out of the very superficial chaos. Thanks to the efficiency of the four men involved any chaos in need of re-ordering was very mild indeed, and Peter had soon been re-ordered to the newly cushioned chair in his bed-sit.

Peter has slept through the day but managed to wake up for long enough to enjoy a leisurely bath before being escorted to his new bed. He seemed somewhat baffled by the luxurious padding on the cot sides but has not made any indication of complaint about the new arrangements. As I was working in the children's room I heard a rattling sound – cot sides? - followed by a clearly enunciated, "Well! Well I never. Well! Well, I never did." But now, at ten minutes to midnight, he is fast asleep and I am beginning to nod-off so I shall end the day and hope that Peter remains restrained in his bed.

Thursday June 18th 2010

I have to report on the outstanding success of Peter's new bed. He, to my great delight and relief, managed to stay in his bed until nine o'clock. The increased amount of sleep has left him feeling totally exhausted and needing to sleep all day. I shall hope that he has not forgotten the essential art of sleeping through the night as well as the day!! More tomorrow.

Friday June 19th 2010

It is most interesting to see the change in Peter's behaviour over these last few days, and most particularly since the arrival of the new bed. The difference may, of course, be entirely coincidental but somehow I feel the most likely factor is the bed. I am also wondering if the fall from our bed on Bank Holiday Monday morning was the result of a mini-stroke. The paramedics checked him for physical damage almost one and a half hours after the fall, so perhaps, after that lapse of time, there was no evidence of anything else. My main point is that the change in behaviour started at that time, and most of the non-activity I had put down to shock. But now I am not so sure. Before the fall he tried, each day, to get out of bed to go to the toilet. This no longer happens, but, of course, the presence of the cot-sides might interfere with the message. He spends the time between half past nine and four o'clock asleep in the chair, which is next to the bed. He then, on waking up, has, over the last three days, tried to get out of the chair so that he can be helped to the bathroom. He enjoys his dinner and then sleeps for another two or three hours before making a close study of his Lever Arch File. You may be interested to know that today, as a result of intense perseverance, Peter managed to make two holes in a cotton handkerchief and fasten the handkerchief into the File. I wonder if he realised the enormity of this achievement. He seems to be a very happy and contented man at the moment. Let us hope it continues.

Saturday June 20th 2010

Today has been a wonderful day as, thanks to Rachel's kindness, I was able to drive to Birmingham and catch up with Paul, Muna, Danny and Alex. Rachel kept an eye on Peter and was required to give the sort of care one would wish not to place on one's children's shoulders! However, she claimed to be able to take such events in her professional stride. Which is, of course, perfectly true but it does not make it any more acceptable to me, as her mother!! Even though Peter has slept during the greater part of today he did emerge as a very helpful person at bath-time. He managed to raise his feet from the ground at the appropriate time and, having accidentally banged his elbow against my head, uttered those immortal words, "Oh, I'm sorry." A bruise is slowly emerging in what is quaintly referred to as the small of his back - where is the large, I wonder - which probably relates back to the rolling out of bed on Bank Holiday Monday. It does not appear to cause him any discomfort so I shall simply wait for it to disappear. I cannot sing the praises of the hospital bed too highly. It is now three minutes past eleven and Peter is comfortably ensconced in his bed, cot sides up and looking most comfortable. I shall finish this paragraph and have a bath, in case this is my night for eight hours sleep. I suspect that most of us have forgotten such a luxury but I am determined to enjoy at least one stretch of eight hours while the brain can still register the experience. You never know, I might find it a practice to be recommended to friends and relations.

Sunday June 21th 2010

I did not quite achieve the eight hours sleep last night, but I did achieve a stupendous six hours. Great is my elation and I shall continue to strive, valiantly, for the eight hour record!! Life seems to be very sedentary and quiet these days. So much so that I am almost finding it unnerving to go into the kitchen and find things just where I left them. I have to say that my folding does not compare with Peter's folding, and my right angles are more than a few degrees short of the mark. However, I do not think Peter is suffering from withdrawal symptoms because he is still able to line up his books on the edge of the bed. Today started rather early because I needed to get Peter up and ready to face the day before I set off for church. The service is now at 10.45am instead of 10.30 am - which is ideal for those of us living some distance away. Rachel called round at midday and found Peter asleep. He was still asleep on my return but I think I shall start the bathing process soon after ten o'clock - in case he feels tired!!

Monday June 22nd 2010

A day of great calm on this Western Front! So I shall leave any further discourse until the district nurse appears tomorrow morning.

Tuesday June 23rd 2010

We have been nudged out of a position of priority and relegated to the bottom of the list!! Our eagerly anticipated visit from the district nurse was cancelled - at very short notice - due to the demands of a departmental meeting. There will, undoubtedly, be another opportunity. Today has, despite the disappointment, been a splendid day. Molly and William were on sparkling form and took great delight in trying to cheat in *Take the Brain*. More news tomorrow - perhaps. I really need to discuss the continence situation with the professionals because it could, I repeat, *could*, have some bearing on what goes on in this house.

Wednesday June 24th 2010

My discourse on the continence situation has been somewhat compromised by the appearance of the district nurse at a time when it was known that I would not be at home. I shall attempt to arrange a further meeting. We remain delighted with the bed and, even if no other promises are realised, I shall count myself as being on a winning wicket. We are not in need of anything else. As the saying goes, 'We are short of nothing we've got!'

I do hope your evening is productive for you, Rachel. Without you my sanity-saving rehearsals with the Police Choir could not take place.

"Very awake tonight. When I arrived Dad had taken up residence on the decorative but fragile wicker table - he was not for moving, but after a brief discussion about Thomas Cranmer he leapt back to his chair. He has drunk almost a whole cup of coffee."

Thank you, Rachel. I am delighted Cranmer has taken over from Cromwell - for the present. Variety is sometimes responsible for enhancing life in a rut!

Thursday June 25th 2010

I suspect there will need to be some close inspection of the routine and perhaps consideration given to extending Peter's opportunities for increased mobility. The thought has left me totally exhausted - so I shall make haste very slowly with the idea - and close for this evening.

Friday June 26th 2010

The implications of Peter's hospital bed.

1. The first and most important result has been a marked improvement in the quality of Peter's sleep. He seems to sleep very quietly, and generally curled up and on his right side. When sleeping in our double bed he preferred to sleep diagonally - until prodded! - uncurled, and on his left side. Has he spent the last forty-seven years in discomfort?????
2. He appears to feel safe and secure in the bed and taps on the cot sides from time to time - perhaps in a questioning way. This morning I discovered that he cannot squeeze through the gap between the end of the cot-side and the foot-end of the bed. I have, as yet, no evidence to support my theory/hope that he cannot climb over the top of the side. At the moment I shall assume that he might be able to climb out if he sets his mind to it.
3. He seems to regard the bed as a daytime coffee table and spends many happy minutes lining up and

straightening his five books, two *English Heritage* magazines and his Lever Arch File. I am relieved to see that he has not forgotten these useful skills.
4. He uses the bed as a prop when trying to stand after straightening the mat by his chair.

These are not wild ramblings but important factors when considering how to make the most of each day, not only for Peter but also for the carer - whichever one of us happens to be on duty!

I am trying to make sure that Peter walks around several times during the day. This seems to be paying off as, on two occasions, Peter has managed to make his way downstairs. Interestingly enough, although I have not seen him coming downstairs yet, I have been encouraged by the careful way he climbs up the stairs. This is somewhat astonishing because only two weeks ago he appeared completely unable to walk without a considerable amount of help. Walking will, I trust, help to reduce the potential for soreness resulting from the incontinence pants. So far his skin is in excellent order.

There will, however, have to be some significant changes in the domestic arrangements.

If he is dressed and taken into the bathroom he is often willing to clean his teeth. After being taken back into the bedroom he is very happy to sit in the chair and allow me to shave him. He will then eat his breakfast and have some coffee. This whole process has probably taken about one hour so he is well and truly exhausted. I have found that he will sleep, doze, wake up, doze, sleep and so on for four or five hours. This period of time should be used carefully, as it may be the only time you can leave him alone with a reasonably clear mind. Calls, visits, shopping, cleaning and gardening are best done at this time of the day.

Again I find it helpful for him to walk about either before or after dinner - which is served between half past five and six o'clock. At some point after dinner he likes to wander around. For the last two days he has found his way downstairs and I have let him stay downstairs for two or three hours. It is important that he climbs the stairs before he becomes too tired.

The message I am receiving - and sending out - is that Peter should not be left unsupervised for more than short periods of time. More thought and organisation will, I am sure, result in finding a responsible and satisfactory way of keeping Peter free to wander when he wishes to, and then staying sitting in his chair when I need him to be sitting down and not wandering. A compromise is all that is necessary.

Another district nurse may call next Wednesday. How wonderful it would be if she could present some idea which would mean that the writing of these pages will not be totally dominated by the demands of the bathroom. But I fear my secret hope is almost certain to be dashed, so I must apologise for the too frequent appearance of the words toilet and toileting. If you are faced with the same situation in your own relationship with Alzheimer's you may be willing and able to overlook the constant repetition. If not . . . what can I say apart from, "Be thankful."

Saturday 27th June 2010

Having decided to follow, without any adjustments, the first stage in my experiment, I took Peter to the toilet as soon as I found him sitting on the end of the bed with his legs wedged between the cot-side end and the foot-end of the bed. This space will, as I mentioned yesterday, not trap his head but it does trap his legs when he tries to toss them over the cot-side. The time was half past eight and so I had to decide to sort Peter out, dress him, help him to clean his teeth, shave his whiskers and then sit him in the chair ready for breakfast. It did not take a major brain to work out that, at that time of the day, it would not have been ideal for me to have been driving to York or Durham - or even attending church or shopping in Sainsbury's. He was ready to face the world by twenty to ten - I was still facing the washing machine. Peter decided against facing the world. Instead he chose to close his eyes and sleep until ten minutes to four - which, according to my calculations, amounts to six hours of soothing sleep. I shall see what happens tomorrow, but I suspect there will be some useful time during the day which can be used for normal living. Most of the evening has been spent resting quietly and/or sleeping. Perhaps the heat has sapped what little energy is left. The only walking has been one short stroll to the toilet.

Sunday June 28th 2010

Today has been very interesting from the routine point of view. Having been alerted to the potential peril of legs becoming wedged at the foot-end of the bed, I was ready for Peter's early morning call! The call came, believe it or not, soon after half past seven. I took him to the toilet and returned him to his bed. At nine o'clock I decided that I would have to wake him up and get him ready to face the day if I had any chance of getting to church on time. However, by ten o'clock Peter was up, washed, dressed, shaved, with teeth cleaned and having had his breakfast and coffee. By five minutes past he was fast asleep in his chair and ready to surface soon after five o'clock. He has managed to walk down the stairs and have his dinner in the Study. He then tidied up the Playmobil in the hall before sitting in the Study and sleeping until ten o'clock. He certainly seems to have recovered some of the ground lost when he fell from the bed, but quite where it leaves us I am not too sure!! At least we have the hospital bed - for which I am most grateful.

Monday June 29th 2010

You will be as astonished as I was to learn that Peter managed, somehow, to climb out of his bed this morning and make his way into his old photographic dark room. I am not certain as to how he managed to leave his bed. Perhaps he vaulted over the cot side or perhaps he managed, against significant odds, to squeeze through the gap between the end of the bed and the end of the cot side. There has been some other evidence of high-level cerebral activity. At one point, during the afternoon, Peter chose a mat from the landing and arranged it, most carefully, next to the bathroom. Having spent the morning asleep he rallied soon after half past three and made his way downstairs. He has spent the rest of the day sleeping, creeping about and arranging the cushion on the rocking chair. This return to some level of activity is more than a little surprising and certainly not what anyone would have expected. It seems very important to me to make the most of these returning skills in order that Peter's life will be a little more varied. The day also seems to be taking some sort of shape so I am feeling very positive about being able to make the most of whatever time becomes available. Not only is there more mobility but there is more in the way of vocalising - even though Peter makes sure that he keeps any sort of meaning to himself! It will be interesting to see how this evolves.

Tuesday June 30th 2010

The first call came at six o'clock when I heard sounds from what is now called Peter's bed-sit. When I went in I found him sitting with his legs wedged between the foot-end and the cot side - he was obviously trying to escape from a bed which was very wet just where he was sitting. Emergency measures were taken and, in almost less than no time, Peter was back in dry clothing and in a dry bed. I went back to bed for half an hour and he went back to sleep. Just before eight o'clock I put the cot side down and went to the surgery to make an appointment for Amber to see one of the doctors. Peter was still fast asleep - and neatly arranged - in bed when I returned.

The next sound of the bed squeaking came soon after half past nine. This time Peter was preparing to get out of bed - which was very good news and excellent timing. By five past ten we had completed the toileting, washing, teeth cleaning, dressing and shaving routine and it was time for breakfast. This was then followed by three hours of sleep.

At half past one I heard a different sound which turned out to be Peter straightening the towels in the bathroom. He was kneeling down but had, most likely, shuffled around on his feet until he reached the bathroom. If I close the doors of the upstairs rooms then there may be the temptation to come downstairs, so I have started to leave the doors open. Maybe he knew he had to walk to the bathroom but then ran out of guidance! Never mind, the shadow of a plan is forming as a result of the behaviour seen so far. Peter had some coffee, an apple and a dinner biscuit before starting on the afternoon's programme of looking at his books and resting. It is now three o'clock and he is asleep - having looked at his books. Who will make the next move?

I am registering, with some interest, that I am feeling much less able to be out of the house now Peter is up and dressed than I did when he was sleeping, freely, in bed until one o'clock in the afternoon.

I am registering, with similar interest, the sincere hope that it will be possible to exchange the current tedium for some exciting seconds in the day. It would be wonderful to be able to reduce the number of times I find myself writing about toileting. That can seem to be more than a little tedious!

At four o'clock Peter has managed to climb downstairs and is busy arranging the furniture - having left four taps running in the kitchen and the utility rooms. I may have mentioned that Norman changed the *measured*-water taps for ordinary lever handle taps, as I suspected that there was rather a lot of water being wasted while waiting for the *measure* to be delivered. It was not possible to stop the flow once it had started - which was not one of the positive features of the system. I am reminded of the saying, "You win some and you lose some" - which is a truth that defies any sort of contradiction.

Has acquiring the hospital bed been a good thing, thus far? To which question I shall respond with a resounding YES - not least because it means I have a bed to myself. Not to mention a room.

It is now fast approaching ten o'clock and Peter should be absolutely exhausted because of the walking about and straightening up of Playmobil characters and vehicles. It is time to bring the day to an end.

Wednesday July 1st 2010

I am starting early in case today is the day when the mists clear and light dawns - for us all. Following a previous plan I lowered the cot side soon after five in the morning - when I happened to wake up. At five past six I heard Peter trying to get out of bed. I took him to the bathroom and managed to fit him into dry pants and pyjama jacket before taking him back to bed. Cot sides up.

At ten in the morning I have lowered the cot side and am ready to catch Peter as soon as he starts to wake up. Today could see the arrival of one of the district nurses. Will this be the beginning of yet another plan of campaign?

I have been reminded of another essential quality in the idea of Keeping Going with your situation. Do not wait for anybody or anything to come along. Make sure you are busy doing something at all times, particularly if it involves sitting in a chair and watching Poirot for the nth time. There is always something you missed last time!!

Peter was ready, willing and able to get up and complete the morning ablutions before eating his breakfast. This all took place between ten forty-five and eleven forty-five. This is helpful, thus far, in preparing a possible timetable. Timetable is possibly a somewhat pretentious term but it is exactly what I mean because, as already mentioned, having some sort of timetable allows for greater flexibility. At least, it does in this house.

I am now considering the idea of putting Peter back into bed after his mid-morning drink and seeing whether he goes back to sleep and stays asleep until noon - or later. This would be better for his posture, it would shorten the day and, selfishly, would allow an extra hour or so for essential jobs - also known as pleasure activities! It is, at present, a consideration and will depend on how many hours Peter is doomed to wander today. This space should be watched!

Another district nurse, Angela, arrived just before three o'clock, but did not need to speak with the patient. Which was as well as he failed to respond but, seemingly, that was of little consequence. Perhaps most things are of little consequence! She left with a promise of a visit by the Continence Team, within the week, who might like to discuss Peter's needs.

It is now half past five in the afternoon and Peter has woken up in order to eat his dinner. I am not quite sure where this leaves my idea of leaving him in bed. Chair or bed? Which shall it be? Which *should* it be? The telling point will come this evening when Rachel will assume the mantle of responsibility.

Thursday July 2nd 2010

Today has been a full and exciting day so there will be a full and exciting report on Friday.

Friday July 3rd 2010

Thursday triumphed because, against considerable odds, all outstanding plans were completed and Joe, Amber and I managed to leave, more or less on time, for our journey to Gawsworth Hall in Cheshire where we were to see a performance of Agatha Christie's *An Unexpected Guest*. This is the sixth year we have attended these wonderful Open Air Theatre Performances by The Green Room Players from nearby Wilmslow. The whole of July is devoted to a wide range of musical, theatrical, vocal, brass band and other talents. The lovely medieval house is open to the audience. Picnics in the grounds are actively encouraged - some people actually bring their own gazebos - and a splendid time is had by all. Last night was no exception. After three weeks of anticipation and organisation we were all able to relax in beautiful surroundings for three hours. It rained throughout most of

Act Two. The audience remained under cover but, as one would expect from an Open Air Theatre, the actors simply carried on as though nothing untoward was happening. Heavy rain at the end did, to some extent, deprive them of a full measure of well-deserved praise. I think their minds, at that point, were on drier things!!

Tony is going to start making the wooden stair gate next Wednesday. I shall also ask him to sort out a suitable bolt for the top of the bathroom door. Turning the water off at the mains has proved to be very simple and straightforward. The only potential for disappointment is when I forget to reconnect the supply. Peter is enjoying sitting in the Study, straightening his socks and clapping his hands. Was there much sense in encouraging Peter to walk after his fall? Of course that depends on your involvement. From my point of view it seems to provide a way of keeping Peter's skin in good order and, we must never forget, there is always the question of the muscle tone. It has resulted in an increase in the carer's workload and, surprisingly, in a considerable outlay of money. Having accepted those factors we are still left with the very real expectation that maintaining a healthy body for as long as possible will reduce work in the long run.

Saturday July 4th 2010

Peter's muscle tone has now reached heights of considerable dizziness. He is managing to lower himself to his knees, straighten any offending mat or incorrectly angled item of furniture, ornament or book. In any other situation I might have suspected him of being a secret student of that excellent example of precision in all matters. I mean, of course Monsieur Hercule Poirot - of Agatha Christie fame. This does, of course, mean that he is able to spend more time out of his chair, which means that his skin stands more chance of staying in good order. I have to admit that this may not be such good news for Rachel when she takes charge during the weekend Joe and I are with Cousin Jean. Two weeks ago the chances of this level of mobility seemed very remote indeed. But, on the positive side, I am certain that if Peter is up, dressed, shaved, with clean teeth and fully breakfasted, then there is an increasing chance of some independent toileting. The day itself has been very good indeed with most things having been accomplished. Tom and I spent just over two hours this morning working on the DVD featuring the Balloon Flight. This was the wonderful occasion when Lillian and I went *Up, Up and Away* in one of Richard Branson's wonderful hot air balloons. This trip was an incredible Christmas gift from the family and proved to be just as thrilling as one could wish it to be. Tom filmed much of the flight and, with great generosity, has undertaken the task of creating a DVD of the whole experience.

Nothing is ever quite as simple as one would like, but I am most impressed with the computer's capacity, under Tom's guidance, to create, store, adjust and file an almost infinite number of tricks. After two hours of diligent recording, checking, repeating, checking again and re-recording, I was astonished to find that we had managed to store a considerable amount of silence. Tom is now wrestling with his hard drive - a successful outcome is guaranteed!

With average luck I will be able to start the bath routine and end the Wanderings of Peter, as he has done more than enough wandering.

Sunday July 5th 2010

Today has been totally different from the last few days. I started the morning routine at nine o'clock, so that Peter would be settled for the day by the time I was ready to go to church at a quarter past ten. I returned soon after midday to find Peter fast asleep in the chair. I remembered to turn on the water before starting the remains of the day! Shortly after two o'clock Peter woke up and I met him, on the landing, en route to the toilet. I had a suspicion that if I left Peter to his own devices he would manage at some level - which might prove to be acceptable. I stayed in the bathroom until I heard the handle of the toilet door being shaken. Peter had managed to pull up the pants but was struggling with the trousers. I am encouraged by this because I am hoping that Peter might be able to manage both items of clothing by the end of the next two weeks - when Joe and I are visiting Cousin Jean. Peter was then happy to go back to his chair and eat an apple and a meal bar - or dinner biscuit. These are easy to eat and he enjoys them. He then went back to sleep until almost six o'clock. He ate his dinner and then spent forty or so minutes moving slowly from room to room. His reflexes are working well in that he is careful to remain in contact with some form of support, be it the wall, a door, or a piece of furniture. I have watched him moving around and have been struck by the care he seems to take when moving from A to B. He was then very happy to kneel down on the floor and spend time straightening the mats, so that they were all correctly placed at right angles to each other. It is now half past nine and Peter is resting in his chair, looking at his Lever Arch File. Why has he made no attempt to come downstairs? What has been different today to cause all this sleeping? Perhaps, by looking carefully at exactly what goes on during the days we shall be in some sort of position to have a modicum of 'control' over what can be organised each day. Today may, of course, be described as a 'one off,' but it may also be a clue as to what might be the shape of the days ahead. Again this is a space to be watched!!

Chapter Six - Another change of direction

Monday July 6th 2010

Thank you for watching this space. Following the morning welcome of the new day, Peter spent the time between half past ten and four o'clock deep in slumber. He then climbed downstairs - carefully, methodically and slowly. Once down I was not certain whether I should shed tears of trepidation - for a further loss of space and time - or give a generous round of applause. I took the easy option and did nothing. The straightening has bordered on the frenetic but, since I have put most things away, there is at least some control over the number of items available for straightening. One improvement is that he has developed a liking for the rocking chair. He has not yet worked out that the curves allowing the rocking cannot be lined up with very much, but he does stay sitting in it for some long while. There has also been a marked increase in the vocalisation. So much so that I am seriously considering whether or not whatever pushed him out of bed, three weeks ago, resulted in a surge of blood to the brain, which is now suddenly capable of more sustained, if somewhat bizarre, behaviour. My plans for developing a routine have not amounted to very much today. So I did what I have always done when my plans are thwarted. Yes, I baked some very large cookies and some large chocolate cakes - also known as brownies. Tom is coming at half past nine tomorrow morning to set up the recording equipment for our second attempt at completing *Up, Up, and Away*. I am afraid Peter is going to have to get in the bath, because I am in danger of being straightened and filed away in a Lever Arch File. For the record I have to note that two Zopiclone sleeping tablets are no more effective than one.

Tuesday July 7th 2010

William was not well enough to attend school today and, as Tom and I had planned to record *Up, Up, and Away*, I was very grateful to Joe for agreeing to start a new holiday job involving William-care for three hours. A good time was had by both boys. Tom and I completed our mission and I, for one, am eagerly awaiting the final outcome! Peter was ready to face the day by half past nine, at which point he closed his eyes and slept until three o'clock - when he woke up in order to eat an apple. Things have been very quiet and orderly and the day has been a happy day because of the presence of Joe, Amber, William and Molly - and I am still a little nearer to sorting out some sort of routine for Peter within the household. Or, possibly, vice versa!!

Wednesday July 8th 2010

It is now almost seven in the evening and Peter has been up and dressed since eleven o'clock. He has, however, spent many of those hours sleeping in his chair in the bedroom. He woke up for his dinner soon after seven and was still upstairs when I left for choir practice. He remained upstairs during Rachel's period of supervision, but came downstairs, most carefully and unaided, within ten minutes of my return at half past nine. Some straightening has taken place but most of the time has been spent in leaving whichever room I happened to be occupying. Companionship is definitely not what he is seeking at the moment. The Playmobil characters are much more interesting. Despite a very swollen right leg, which has resulted from a big bruise he sustained when he knocked his leg two weeks ago, he seems to be very comfortable kneeling on the floor and lining up the figures. Tomorrow is the day when the substantial stair gate will be made and fitted. Tony, Mark's friendly handyman, is coming to sort it all out in the morning. My hope is that, by the time Joe and I travel south, all safety measures will be in place, so that Rachel is not left with too many challenges of an unexpected nature. Although, as we well know, some will have escaped our attention!

Thursday July 9th 2010

Today has been cancelled, binned, disposed of, whatever you like to use as a passive verb, due to compassion fatigue.

I have just retrieved part of it to say that Tony has built the new gate and I have just finished putting on the second coat of paint. It will be excellent, as will the lock on the bathroom door.

Friday July 10th 2010

Today has been a much better day for all people involved in it. The new gate received its third coat of paint this morning and has already proved its superior strength and resistance. I am still not entirely comfortable with the prospect of Peter being condemned to wandering round the upstairs rooms. Not because of a problem with the rooms but I feel there is not a great deal of space for wandering. I know it is the right decision because Peter found climbing the stairs very difficult indeed last night. So much so that I thought it might be impossible to climb those three stairs on the turn of the landing. In the end, with my head pushing into his back and with my right arm trying to instil some sort of sense into his right leg, we did manage those last few steps. He pointed over the gate this afternoon as if to suggest it might be a good idea to wander downstairs. So I simply said, "No, the door has been closed." This was always my response when he was trying to escape from the house by means of the front door. He seemed to accept it then and, to my great relief, appeared to accept it today. We are still managing to get in and out of the bath, but it is not an easy manoeuvre for anybody. At present I am not certain what I will introduce as the next stage. I am currently sitting in Peter's bed-sit, but am planning on moving out soon as I am obviously invading his space - such as it is. Ah well! We can only try.

Saturday July 11th 2010

A good day was further redeemed by the arrival of Molly and William for their 'sleep-over.' This always guarantees a very happy time for all active participants. They are wonderful guests because their great determination in life is to play together and enjoy themselves!

Sunday July 12th 2010

Now the security of the wooden gate has been tested, inspected and accepted as part of the surroundings, I am using the opportunity to make some further assessment as to what Peter is able to do, when I am not physically present, as far as his mobility is concerned. I can hear and work out a lot of his movements if I stay at the bottom of the stairs - carefully tuned in to every sound, be it a creaking floorboard or a shuffling footstep, although these are more difficult to gauge on the carpet!! He is capable of making his slow way onto the landing and then round and into the toilet. He can kneel down and straighten the waterproof mats which cover the Axminster carpeting and he can get up from his chair and sit down in the chair. He can get off the bed and sit on the edge of the bed. He cannot, as yet, swing his legs back onto the bed. I say as yet, because, as I have already mentioned, none of us could have anticipated this level of regained mobility.

This mobility is not of a random nature but is very closely connected with reasons.

1. Getting off the bed is obviously confined to the getting up process. This is, I suspect, a response to the bladder, but, although he recognises the toilet, he appears to have no recollection of what it is for.
2. Again he only gets out of the chair when responding to the same urge. He pulls himself along using the wall and anything else he can hold onto. It is fascinating to see how he uses instinctive movements as a means of self-protection. He will get out of the chair on two occasions during the time he is not in bed. Straightening activities are confined to these occasions but can last for several minutes.
3. He returns to his chair independently if he cannot see me. If I make myself visible he seems to lose the ability to move under his own steam!!!
4. Getting out of the chair last thing at night is unpredictable - as is making a sensible attempt at sitting on the edge of the bed before I can swing his legs round.

5. Getting Peter in and out of the bath is always a matter of good luck. All the time he can remember to bend his knee and hold onto the rails, we are in business. Also we do not need too many repeats of forgetting how to sit down in the bath. Sometimes a discreet push is necessary! I am still not quite certain of how I shall

arrange an alternative to sitting in the bath for twenty minutes.

All this mobility, be it spontaneous or enforced, has to be improving his circulation - not forgetting the all-important muscle tone. It is worth recording this tedious material for the next few days, in case some little nugget seems to be relevant when Rachel assumes the Mantle of Responsibility this coming weekend.

Monday July 13th 2010

Today has been an excellent day with Peter managing to totter around the bedroom, look out of the window, straighten the wicker basket containing his bedding and to unscrew the black knob on the cot side. It is the knob one has to pull in or out in order to lower the left hand side of the cot. I have never seen him show any interest in the knob, neither did I know he was aware of its existence, as it is scarcely visible to those of us searching for it at the end of the day!!

Tuesday July 14th 2010.

I cannot put too much emphasis on the importance of leaving Peter to do things in his own time - and, very occasionally, in his own way. This is, I realise, particularly important as far as toileting is concerned. Now he is walking with more confidence it is safe to leave him to totter to the toilet, during the daytime, when he considers it necessary.

Tuesday July 21st 2010

Peter has slept throughout most of the day. One new development, which I am advised is entirely normal at this stage in the disease, is a concentration on feeling the skin on the palm of his hand. Peter feels the skin on the palms of both hands in a routine and alternating sequence.

Wednesday July 22nd 2010

Another peaceful and silent day with Peter keeping the drama for the time I was out at choir practice. At that particular point he decided to straighten up the mats so that, when Rachel arrived, he had straightened the mats and was busy trying to arrange himself alongside one of the mats on the floor. Somehow, after forty minutes skilful manoeuvring - not to mention the aid of the slatted bath seat - Rachel, with truly consummate skill, managed to ease Peter into his own chair. The whole exercise had proved to be most exhausting and he had to fall asleep within minutes of placing himself in the chair. I did not hear about Rachel's exhaustion and overwhelming need for sleep - naturally. . .

Thursday July 23rd 2010

I have been glancing over my notes and the kaleidoscopic view of the progress of the disease, and find myself being astonished by the change in Peter since the end of May. He has lost a great deal in the way of mobility and the ability to show recognition of the presence of people, food, drink and even sounds. But he has hung on to other elements. For example there was an occasion this evening when he fell onto his knees. While kneeling on the floor he tried to straighten two mats before beginning to shuffle and crawl on his knees halfway across the bedroom until he reached the edge of the bed. I was watching through the doorway to see exactly what he was able to do. It seemed to me that he was following some basic instincts or reflexes which enabled him to crawl and then pull himself into a semi-standing position. As he could lean against the substantial side of the bed he was then able to manoeuvre himself onto the bed itself. The whole process took rather less than ten minutes. I was left with the firm idea that, had I intervened at any stage, I would have interrupted a flow - possibly a slow flow - of messages from his brain to his body and he would not have been able to complete the exercise of finding his feet and being able to get as far as the bed and sit down. If a body is not hurt it may well be able to find a possible way of getting out of trouble. Toddlers try and do it all the time! This great spurt of activity came after a six hour sleep following the normal morning activities: perfunctory washing, cleaning teeth, dressing, shaving and eating breakfast. Dinner appeared at six o'clock after which the mat straightening commenced. This followed for the usual twenty or thirty minutes before he went back to sleep in the chair. Bed time began soon after eleven o'clock and finished, with Peter in bed, at a quarter to midnight. The present routine has become reasonably well established and presents few problems.

I do hope there are no other changes lurking in the shadows as this routine, although not quite as flexible as the previous routine - because Peter does require rather more supervision now - is very manageable and he is certainly very peaceful. Many are the benefits of plentiful periods of sleep - for all concerned. It also makes loving and cherishing so much easier!

Chapter Seven - The Unravelling

Thursday September 30th 2010

Some remarkable changes proved to have been lurking in the shadows!! You may have noted the date of this entry and perhaps have started to wonder what has caused the eight week lapse. I have missed the opportunity to try and make sense of each day's experiences and now finally find myself looking forward to sorting out some of the events of the last few weeks.

Tuesday October 12th 2010

How extraordinary! I can see what may be the only way of putting a full stop at the end of this particular phase in life. It had seemed, at one point, to be a simple enough process to write about what happened on Friday July 24th. Now, however, it may be more appropriate to state, simply and succinctly, what happened on that day. Seven o'clock in the morning saw emergency arrangements for me to be taken into hospital and for suitable and appropriate accommodation to be found for Peter. Thanks to the Quick Response Team - namely Rachel and Mark - an ideal place was found for him at The Vicarage Care Home in Audenshaw, where he continues to live a peaceful and seemingly contented life. After undergoing major surgery I was diagnosed with a malignant Brenner ovarian cancer on

September 17th, and arrangements were then made for six months of chemotherapy treatment to commence in mid-October. I am hoping to be given a clean bill of health by Summer 2011.

Our responsibility for Peter is to ensure that he has a visit from one member of the family each and every day. Peter's care has been taken out of our hands and placed in the hands of the staff at The Vicarage. Our responsibility for visiting is, as far as I can see, particularly important, as the fact that Peter does not recognise or remember any of us makes regular visits even more vital. It is, perhaps, the only way we can preserve any sense of identity for Peter.

In conclusion it may be worth mentioning that, although our family has experienced an extremely close and intimate relationship with Alzheimer's disease, it will be one that is unlikely to have been repeated, in its entirety, by any other family. This is, of course, because all experiences will be different and pertinent only to each individual family. But, and it is a very big but, real awareness and the consequent understanding of the many facets of this disease, will only be possible when those caring families living with the complexities of Alzheimer's disease can join forces, through recounting and sharing their own experiences, and painting the picture on a suitably large canvas.

Armed with this material the experts will be in a much better position to begin to comprehend the incomprehensible.

Perhaps *you* are the person to do this job. Perhaps *your* journey has equipped you to see beyond the mundane elements of the caring role. Perhaps *you* have a vision that will inspire others and make the voice of such a great army of carers heard in places where it can bring about some real and positive change.

Chapter Eight - Crossroads

I had always regarded Crossroads as being times or spaces in life where it would be possible to continue to exercise one's individual preference or choice of direction. After all, in theory, the options are simple. North, South, East or West or even Left, Right, Straight on or, on occasions, Go back. What we may not be prepared for are the crossroads which have barriers across each exit, thus making it impossible for us to have any real influence on making a personal decision.

Knowing that I am talking with people who have an intimate understanding of the many and varied consequences on family, and family life, when Alzheimer's disease takes its relentless hold on a dearly loved family member, I feel certain that you will, each one of you, have arrived at the second set of crossroads - the ones with the four barriers. We don't always see these barriers but we know they are there after we have hit them. This may sound somewhat negative but, in some situations, those blocked crossroads may prove to be positive and life saving.

This has certainly been true in my situation. After ten years spent caring for Peter, including two years with double incontinence, severe mobility problems and feeding problems - which arose when Peter could not feed himself and had lost the mechanism which told him whether or not he was hungry - I thought I had got things sorted out - to my satisfaction at least.

Our big bedroom had become what we called Peter's Bed-Sit.

A hospital bed had been installed, his favourite chair had been fitted with a rising mechanism - which made moving him in and out of the chair so much easier and, best of all, I had mastered the art of shaving him with a Gillette wet razor without cutting his skin or knocking his nose. Everything seemed to be going along in a reasonable fashion. My daughter, living in Denton, and my younger son - living in Marple Bridge - supplied me with every possible support - including the ability to laugh at the many ridiculous elements presented by life, while my older son, in Birmingham, had his own witty and much appreciated philosophy which helped us all to keep our heads above water. I could wake up each morning feeling that I could manage today - and if I had enjoyed more than four hours sleep then I would manage brilliantly. You note I have still retained my modesty! I had even made two enquiries about care for Peter should I be prevented, for whatever reason, from being responsible for his full time care.

On the evening of July 23rd 2010, I wrote, in the journal I was keeping on Peter's journey along the Alzheimer's Road:

"Everything seems to be on an even keel at present. All is manageable. I hope there is nothing sinister lurking round the corner. It is now two o'clock in the morning and I am going to bed."

At that point all crossroads seemed open - although, to be honest, I had spent more time than I was prepared to admit, curled up with a hot water bottle trying to relieve the severe abdominal pains which seemed to have taken a hold on me. But that is all hindsight - along with its wisdom.

The barriers appeared, three hours later, at half past five in the morning when I was awakened by Peter who, contrary to all ideas and expectations, had managed to escape from his hospital bed - complete with cot sides - and was standing in the doorway of the room in which I was sleeping. He was wet through. The crossroads were still open because I was able to put him on the toilet, strip the bed, take the bedding downstairs, set the washing machine running, go back upstairs, remake his bed, sort Peter out, put him back into bed and secure the cot-side. I then took the crossroad which should have taken me back to bed in the children's room where I was sleeping. It was at that precise moment that the barriers appeared. Try as I would I could neither sit, stand, lie down, curl up or do anything in comfort. Added to which I was alternately shivering with cold or feeling very hot and clammy, with both conditions being accompanied by intense and violent shaking. I could, and did, make one choice - which would be the last for many, many weeks. I picked up the phone, rang my daughter and said four words I have never, at any time, said to anybody. "I am not well."

I had reached the Major Crossroads, which were barred in all four directions. Barred to me, that is, but open to other people who were able to make plans and wise decisions on my behalf. Decisions which I, with the arrogance that comes with thinking that I was the only person capable of looking after Peter, would have been incapable of making.

For the next six months people or circumstances told me what to do, when to do it and even how to do it. During this time I received such wonderful support in the form of love, prayers, kind thoughts, good wishes, laughter and compassion that eventually I was able to find another set of crossroads - with access to one or two choices.

I realised, when I was eventually able to see Peter that the care he was receiving from The Vicarage was better than anything I could offer. He did not know me, but he had not known me for the previous four years. He only sensed that he was safe and, I hope, that he was loved and cherished.

With so much support I would not have dared to fail to respond to the treatment and get better. I have to accept the fact that I will not be able to care for Peter at home, but I have also realised that the barriers have been removed from the crossroads and I can, for good or ill, make my own decisions - provided, I might add, that they fit in with what everybody else has already decided. So my last words today will have to be: Know when to stop and, perhaps suspect, as I do, that your God is on crossroad duty at all times - He may even be The Crossroads.

It is now the eleventh day of September 2014 and I have just returned from my daily visit to Peter in The Vicarage Care Home. The Vicarage has been everything I could have desired for Peter. He has been treated with great compassion, dignity and respect over these last four and a half years, by such kind and professional staff who really do treat all the residents as important family members. Peter has been confined to his bed for twenty-fours hours of each day for the last two and a half years, bereft of speech or any means of communication, unable to move to a comfortable position, should he so wish, and chained to a body with no element of independence. He is spoon-fed with food prepared to the consistency of a fairly thick custard and has thickened fruit juice to drink, often from a spoon. It is impossible to place oneself in such a situation and claim to understand how it must feel to be the Peter who occupies that physical body in that particular bed - comfortable as it may seem.

It is important not to lose sight of the fact that Peter is still the man we love and cherish. It is my profound hope that the world of dementia, in which he has lived for so long, is as peaceful and calm for him as his behaviour - for want of a better word - would appear to suggest. Mercifully he no longer becomes agitated or frightened but seems to spread a feeling of calm and acceptance. I could not quite bring myself to write the word contentment, but my final thought is that, as a man of faith, Peter may already be at peace with his God.

We have no knowledge of the time our relationship with Alzheimer's disease will come to an end, but there is one important aspect of our present lives that Alzheimer's disease - that enemy at the gate - cannot control. We have our own memories of the one we are loving and cherishing. This means that we can, and possibly must, dream and reminisce for two instead of one. This may be all that is needed to connect that lonely soul with its forgotten body with dignity and integrity. Alzheimer's disease has not always dominated our lives so we should not allow it to take too big a hold now. We are the carers and will continue to care, and to love and to cherish.

Thank you for your companionship on this stretch of the road. I wish you peace and every blessing in all that you do and the strength to continue your own journey, as I shall hope to continue mine.

For Your Own Notes

For Your Own Notes

Made in the USA
Charleston, SC
07 April 2015